GALACTIC RESPIRA

GALACTIC RESPIRA

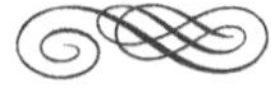

Nebulizer Nebula Symphony

HURMUZ AIN

Spectra Enterprise

Contents

Table Of Content   1

Introduction   3

Chapter 1   6

Chapter 2   17

Chapter 3   28

Chapter 4   42

Chapter 5   58

Chapter 6   73

Chapter 7   89

Chapter 8   104

Chapter 9   117

Table Of Content

Introduction

Chapter 1: Celestial Prelude
1.1 Introduction to the protagonist, a character struggling with respiratory issues.
1.2 Discovery of the Nebula Symphony, a groundbreaking nebulizer technology.
1.3 The promise of a cosmic journey toward respiratory relief.

Chapter 2: Breath of Nebulae
2.1 Protagonist's first encounter with the Galactic Respira device.
2.2 Description of the nebula-inspired mist and its soothing effects.
2.3 Initial skepticism and the gradual acceptance of its therapeutic potential.

Chapter 3: Astral Diagnosis
3.1 Medical examination and diagnosis of the protagonist's respiratory condition.
3.2 Introduction to the medical professionals and their collaboration with Nebula Symphony technology.
3.3 Unveiling the science behind the celestial healing process.

Chapter 4: Nebula Alchemy
4.1 Explanation of the nebulization process and the celestial elements used in the Symphony.
4.2 Protagonist's journey through the transformational alchemy of the Nebula Symphony.
4.3 Gradual improvement in respiratory health and the emergence of hope.

Chapter 5: Cosmic Challenges
5.1 Introduction of obstacles and challenges faced by the protagonist on the path to recovery.

5.2 External skepticism and societal barriers to accepting Nebula Symphony as a legitimate treatment.

5.3 Protagonist's determination to overcome challenges and continue the celestial journey.

Chapter 6: Nebula's Guidance

6.1 Discovery of a mentor figure or guide who helps the protagonist navigate the cosmic healing process.

6.2 Spiritual and emotional support provided by the Nebula Symphony community.

6.3 Developing a deeper connection with the nebula-inspired therapy.

Chapter 7: Galactic Harmony

7.1 Protagonist's integration into the Nebula Symphony community and the formation of bonds with fellow users.

7.2 Collaborative efforts to promote awareness and acceptance of the Galactic Respira technology.

7.3 Celebration of small victories and shared success stories.

Chapter 8: Celestial Resilience

8.1 Unexpected setbacks and challenges that test the protagonist's resilience.

8.2 The role of Nebula Symphony in fostering emotional and mental well-being.

8.3 Protagonist's determination to persevere through difficulties.

Chapter 9: Cosmic Transformation

9.1 Protagonist's complete transformation both physically and emotionally.

9.2 Reflection on the journey and personal growth experienced throughout the Nebula Symphony therapy.

9.3 Acknowledgment of the galactic symphony as a catalyst for positive change.

Introduction

In the tremendous breadth of clinical development and helpful headways, the convergence of innovation and recuperating has birthed a peculiarity that rises above the customary and wanders into the divine domains of help. Enter the Cosmic Respira: Nebulizer Cloud Orchestra, an exceptional wonder that wires state of the art innovation with the infinite motivation drawn from the profundities of the universe.

The human experience is complicatedly laced with the cadence of breath, the inward breath and exhalation that supports life itself. However, for some people, this fundamental demonstration turns into a battle, a fight against respiratory sicknesses that reduce the personal satisfaction and cutoff ordinary exercises. The Cloud Orchestra arises as an encouraging sign in this battle, a divine ensemble intended to fit with the human respiratory framework and achieve a groundbreaking flood of help.

Beginnings of Heavenly Mending

The beginning of this grandiose mending venture lies in the juncture of logical request and heavenly marvel. As specialists dug into the complexities of respiratory treatment, they looked for motivation past traditional techniques. The divine scene of clouds, with their ethereal fogs and infinite appeal, started an inventive way to deal with mending innovation.

Drawing from the loftiness of these enormous peculiarities, the Cloud Orchestra was considered. Its plan impersonates the charming fog developments tracked down in clouds, changing clinical vapor sprayers into a mitigating and helpful experience. The ensemble coordinates a sensitive harmony between science and workmanship, implanting the mending system with a vast stylish that reverberates with clients on a significant level.

Divulging the Cloud Orchestra

At the core of this progressive remedial methodology lies the Cosmic Respira gadget, the conductor through which the Cloud Orchestra shows signs of life. The gadget cleverly changes over restorative mixtures into a cloud propelled fog, conveying a fine and designated spray for inward breath. This fog, much the same as the grandiose pith tracked down in clouds, saturates the respiratory framework, venturing profound into the lungs with a delicate yet strong impact.

The orchestra unfurls as the fog fits with the body's breathing musicality, embracing every inward breath and exhalation with a divine rhythm. This synchronization isn't just an actual interaction; a vivid encounter rises above the clinical domain, offering clients a feeling of association with the enormous dance of the universe.

Connecting Science and Serenity

Installed inside the Cloud Ensemble's divine charm is a vigorous logical establishment. Broad exploration, careful testing, and cooperative endeavors among clinical specialists and mechanical trailblazers have finished in a treatment that weds viability with style.

The airborne prescription conveyed by the Cosmic Respira gadget is custom-made to address a horde of respiratory sicknesses, from constant circumstances to intense episodes. Its accuracy focusing on guarantees ideal ingestion and viability, while the cloud propelled fog calms and solaces, giving an all encompassing way to deal with respiratory wellbeing.

However, past its clinical viability, the Cloud Ensemble's actual power lies in its capacity to rise above the domain of simple treatment. It wanders into the domain of serenity, offering clients actual help as well as a psychological and profound desert garden in the midst of the tumult of wellbeing challenges.

Embracing the Inestimable Excursion

As people set out on their Cloud Orchestra venture, they cross a vast scene of mending and disclosure. Every breath turns into a tribute to divine concordance, a bit nearer to recovering a feeling of business as usual and imperativeness. Inside this excursion, clients find a local area joined by shared encounters, supporting each other through the preliminaries and wins of respiratory wellbeing.

The Cloud Orchestra isn't simply a clinical development; it's an inestimable buddy on the way to better respiratory wellbeing. Its ethereal fog and divine reverberation welcome clients to embrace an excursion past treatment — a journey that resounds with the vast ensemble of the actual universe.

Cosmic Respira: Nebulizer Cloud Orchestra remains as a demonstration of the resourcefulness of human development propelled by the greatness of the universe. It rises above the limits of customary treatment, offering mending as well as a vivid encounter that interlaces science with heavenly miracle.

In the parts that follow, we'll dig further into the multi-layered features of this grandiose excursion. We'll investigate the individual stories of people whose lives have been changed by the Cloud Ensemble, analyze the logical complexities behind its viability, and praise the solidarity encouraged inside its dynamic local area. Get ready to set out on an infinite odyssey — one where the limits between innovation, recuperating, and the universe obscure into an orchestra of heavenly health.

Chapter 1

Celestial Prelude

In the tremendous breadth of clinical development and helpful headways, the convergence of innovation and recuperating has birthed a peculiarity that rises above the customary and wanders into the divine domains of help. Enter the Cosmic Respira: Nebulizer Cloud Orchestra, an exceptional wonder that wires state of the art innovation with the infinite motivation drawn from the profundities of the universe.

The human experience is complicatedly laced with the cadence of breath, the inward breath and exhalation that supports life itself. However, for some people, this fundamental demonstration turns into a battle, a fight against respiratory sicknesses that reduce the personal satisfaction and cutoff ordinary exercises. The Cloud Orchestra arises as an encouraging sign in this battle, a divine ensemble intended to fit with the human respiratory framework and achieve a groundbreaking flood of help.

Beginnings of Heavenly Mending

The beginning of this grandiose mending venture lies in the juncture of logical request and heavenly marvel. As specialists dug into the complexities of respiratory treatment, they looked for motivation past traditional techniques. The divine scene of clouds, with their ethereal fogs and infinite appeal, started an inventive way to deal with mending innovation.

Drawing from the loftiness of these enormous peculiarities, the Cloud Orchestra was considered. Its plan impersonates the charming fog developments tracked down in clouds, changing clinical vapor sprayers into a mitigating and helpful experience. The ensemble coordinates a sensitive harmony between science and workmanship, implanting the mending system with a vast stylish that reverberates with clients on a significant level.

Divulging the Cloud Orchestra

At the core of this progressive remedial methodology lies the Cosmic Respira gadget, the conductor through which the Cloud Orchestra shows signs of life. The gadget cleverly changes over restorative mixtures into a cloud propelled fog, conveying a fine and designated spray for inward breath. This fog, much the same as the grandiose pith tracked down in clouds, saturates the respiratory framework, venturing profound into the lungs with a delicate yet strong impact.

The orchestra unfurls as the fog fits with the body's breathing musicality, embracing every inward breath and exhalation with a divine rhythm. This synchronization isn't just an actual interaction; a vivid encounter rises above the clinical domain, offering clients a feeling of association with the enormous dance of the universe.

Connecting Science and Serenity

Installed inside the Cloud Ensemble's divine charm is a vigorous logical establishment. Broad exploration, careful testing, and cooperative endeavors among clinical specialists and mechanical trailblazers have finished in a treatment that weds viability with style.

The airborne prescription conveyed by the Cosmic Respira gadget is custom-made to address a horde of respiratory sicknesses, from constant circumstances to intense episodes. Its accuracy focusing on guarantees ideal ingestion and viability, while the cloud propelled fog calms and solaces, giving an all encompassing way to deal with respiratory wellbeing.

However, past its clinical viability, the Cloud Ensemble's actual power lies in its capacity to rise above the domain of simple treatment. It wanders into the domain of serenity, offering clients actual help as well as a psychological and profound desert garden in the midst of the tumult of wellbeing challenges.

Embracing the Inestimable Excursion

As people set out on their Cloud Orchestra venture, they cross a vast scene of mending and disclosure. Every breath turns into a tribute to divine concordance, a bit nearer to recovering a feeling of business as usual and imperativeness. Inside this excursion, clients find a local area joined by shared encounters, supporting each other through the preliminaries and wins of respiratory wellbeing.

The Cloud Orchestra isn't simply a clinical development; it's an inestimable buddy on the way to better respiratory wellbeing. Its ethereal fog and divine reverberation welcome clients to embrace an excursion past treatment — a journey that resounds with the vast ensemble of the actual universe.

Cosmic Respira: Nebulizer Cloud Orchestra remains as a demonstration of the resourcefulness of human development propelled by the greatness of the universe. It rises above the limits of customary treatment, offering mending as well as a vivid encounter that interlaces science with heavenly miracle.

In the parts that follow, we'll dig further into the multi-layered features of this grandiose excursion. We'll investigate the individual stories of people whose lives have been changed by the Cloud Ensemble, analyze the logical complexities behind its viability, and praise the solidarity encouraged inside its dynamic local area. Get ready to set out on an infinite odyssey — one where the limits between innovation, recuperating, and the universe obscure into an orchestra of heavenly health.

1.1 Introduction to the protagonist, a character struggling with respiratory issues.

In the rambling universe of Cosmic Respira: Nebulizer Cloud Orchestra, the core of the story beats with the presentation of a hero whose life is complicatedly woven with the sensitive strings of respiratory battles. This character fills in as the focal point through which the peruser witnesses the extraordinary force of the Cloud Orchestra, a divine song promising comfort and revival.

The hero rises out of the story shadows as a figure wrestling with the significant ramifications of respiratory difficulties. Every breath, once underestimated, turns into a demonstration of the delicacy of life and the persevering battle against an inconspicuous enemy. The initial sections of this inestimable excursion paint a piercing representation of weakness, as the hero stands up to the everyday ensemble of wheezes and pants, a cacophonous song repeating the battle for breath.

As the story unfurls, layers of the hero's life are carefully stripped away, uncovering a complicated embroidery of encounters formed by the relentless hit the dance floor with respiratory restrictions. The peruser is brought into the hero's reality, feeling the heaviness of each and every worked breath and the profound cost claimed by the tenacious ghost of windedness. This presentation isn't only a work of clinical subtleties; it is an encouragement to feel for the human behind the illness, to perceive the strength inside weakness.

The hero's day to day everyday practice, once unremarkable, turns into a combat zone against the limitations forced by respiratory difficulties. Everyday undertakings change into Considerable accomplishments as the hero wrestles with the polarity of a body longing for air and a soul longing for freedom. The battle turns into a quiet, personal discussion between the hero and the universe, a discourse set apart by the musical inward breath and exhalation that characterizes the human experience.

Inside the domain of this battle, the Cloud Orchestra arises as a divine commitment — a supernatural tune that holds the possibility to fit with the conflicting notes of respiratory misery. The hero, troubled by the heaviness of restrictions, projects a watchful look toward this inestimable intercession, distrustful yet confident that the Cloud Orchestra might offer the way to opening the shackles of windedness.

The story investigation of the hero's inward world is an excursion into the profound subtleties of living with respiratory difficulties. Dissatisfaction, sadness, and snapshots of calm acknowledgment make a multicolored close to home scene. Perusers are welcome to feel the hero's longing for predictability, to reverberate with the quiet weeps for freedom that reverberation in each stressed breath.

This presentation rises above the limits of a simple clinical conclusion; it wanders into the domain of the human soul, depicting the hero as a strong soul exploring a universe of difficulties. The Cloud Ensemble, covered in vast charm, becomes a remedial gadget as well as an encouraging sign, a far off star promising a respite from the gravitational draw of respiratory requirements.

The hero's relationship with their own body turns into a point of convergence, a powerful interaction between actual impediments and the interminable longing for a breath unrestricted by the chains of respiratory misery. The Cloud Orchestra, floating on the outskirts of the hero's mindfulness, represents the potential for a groundbreaking collaboration — a divine organization among innovation and the human soul.

As the hero wrestles with the recurring pattern of respiratory difficulties, the Cloud Orchestra steadily moves from the edges of attention to the front of thought. Its divine charm turns into an attractive power, bringing the hero into an inestimable dance of probability. The hero's underlying suspicion dances with a developing interest, foretelling the inestimable odyssey looking for them as they step onto the way cleared by the Cloud Ensemble.

The peruser turns into a compassionate observer to the hero's excursion, exploring the maze of feelings that go with the everyday showdown with respiratory impediments. It is an excursion set apart by the piercing convergence of weakness and strength, as the hero faces the truth of their condition while gripping to the dauntless soul that won't be doused.

In the rich embroidery of the hero's presentation, the Cloud Orchestra isn't simply a mechanical wonder; it is a grandiose partner in the hero's mission for breath and freedom. The account, implanted with compassion and subtlety, allures the peruser to set out on this heavenly odyssey, to remain close by the hero at the junction of weakness and versatility, and to expect the groundbreaking crescendo that anticipates in the sections that follow.

1.2 Discovery of the Nebula Symphony, a groundbreaking nebulizer technology.
Inside the grandiose embroidery of Cosmic Respira: Nebulizer Cloud Orchestra, a crucial second unfurls — the revelation of a weighty nebulizer innovation that vows to rethink the scene of respiratory wellbeing. This part denotes a heavenly crossroads where the domains of development and recuperating combine, pushing the story into unknown regions of inestimable help.

The story unfurls against the setting of the hero's respiratory battles, an ensemble of heaves and wheezes that highlights the criticalness for extraordinary mediation. As though directed by the inestimable flows themselves, the hero coincidentally finds the Cloud Ensemble — an ethereal commitment epitomized inside the smooth plan of the Cosmic Respira gadget. The disclosure turns into an epochal second, a fortunate arrangement of grandiose powers and human need.

The Cosmic Respira gadget, with its cloud propelled style, entices like a heavenly alarm, promising an amicable mix of mechanical accuracy and vast motivation. The hero's most memorable experience with this extraordinary device is a tactile encounter, as though breathing in the actual pith of clouds — a divine fog that holds the possibility to disseminate the shadows cast by respiratory difficulties.

The Cloud Ensemble, at its center, is in excess of a mechanical wonder; it is a heavenly director organizing an orchestra of recuperating. As the hero likely draws in with the Cosmic Respira gadget, a delicate fog suggestive of cloud developments wraps their faculties. It is an instinctive association with the infinite, an inward breath of heavenly commitment that rises above the clinical limits of conventional respiratory treatments.

The section unfurls as the Cloud Orchestra becomes the dominant focal point, disclosing its progressive way to deal with nebulization. Clinical sprayers, once bound to the domain of clinical productivity, go through a transformation inside the Cosmic Respira gadget. The speculative chemistry of this nebulizer innovation changes restorative mixtures into a cloud motivated fog, a fragile dance of particles that reflects the inestimable expressive dance of the actual universe.

The peruser is drenched in the complex subtleties of this nebulization cycle, a union of science and heavenly style. The Cloud Orchestra turns into a scaffold between the minute domain of clinical mediation and the plainly visible magnificence of the universe. The fog, injected with the quintessence of clouds, turns into a course for mending — a heavenly mixture that navigates the respiratory scene with artfulness and accuracy.

The Cosmic Respira gadget, as the vessel for this groundbreaking fog, turns into a seal of creativity and sympathy. Its plan isn't only practical yet reminiscent, drawing motivation from the divine ponders that decorate the night sky. The hero's connection with this nebulizer innovation is likened to a divine fellowship, a second where the limits between the human and the inestimable haze into an amicable entirety.

The Cloud Orchestra, as a momentous nebulizer innovation, rises above the impediments of regular respiratory treatments. Its accuracy focusing on guarantees that the restorative fog arrives at the most profound openings of the lungs, where the inestimable dance of mending happens. The hero turns into a member in this heavenly movement, breathing in the cloud propelled fog with every breath — a musical fellowship with the actual substance of the universe.

The innovation's viability isn't just a demonstration of its logical establishment yet additionally a tribute to the marriage of craftsmanship and recuperating. The Cloud Ensemble acquaints a tangible aspect with respiratory treatment, changing the demonstration of inward breath into a multisensory experience. The hero's excursion with the Cosmic Respira gadget isn't only a clinical interaction yet a journey through an inestimable orchestra that reverberates with the actual embodiment of being.

As the hero's respiratory scene goes through a transformation, so does their impression of the Cloud Orchestra. Distrust, inborn despite novel treatments, gives way to a developing acknowledgment of the groundbreaking expected inside the vast fog. The Cosmic Respira gadget turns into a confided in partner, an encouraging sign in the beforehand unfamiliar domains of respiratory help.

The story unfurls with a sensitive dance between the hero and the Cloud

Ensemble, as trust blooms and the mending venture picks up speed. The peruser is brought into the hero's insight, feeling the rhythmic movement of grandiose fog, and seeing the unobtrusive changes in their physical and close to home prosperity. The Cosmic Respira gadget isn't simply an instrument; it turns into an infinite friend, an aide through the neglected systems of respiratory wellbeing.

The Cloud Orchestra's earth shattering nature reaches out past its nearby effect on the hero. It resonates through the clinical scene, rocking the boat of respiratory treatments. Clinical experts, after seeing the extraordinary impacts, become pioneers in supporting for the combination of Cloud Orchestra innovation into standard respiratory consideration. The revelation takes on an aggregate importance, promising a change in outlook in the way to deal with respiratory wellbeing on a worldwide scale.

In the embroidery of disclosure, the Cloud Ensemble arises as a divine beacon, directing the hero as well as a whole local area toward the shores of respiratory prosperity. The noteworthy nebulizer innovation turns into an impetus for discussions around development, openness, and the crossing point of science and compassion in medical care.

The peruser, enchanted by the grandiose charm of the Cloud Orchestra, is welcome to observe a mechanical leap forward as well as a renaissance in respiratory consideration. The Cosmic Respira gadget turns into a figurative key, opening the vast doors to a domain where respiratory battles are met with empathy, development, and the groundbreaking force of the heavenly. In this part of disclosure, the Cloud Ensemble stands up for itself as an encouraging sign — an enormous disclosure that proclaims the beginning of another period in respiratory health.

The revelation of the Cloud Orchestra, a notable nebulizer innovation, spreads out a divine embroidery woven with development, trust, and the commitment of extraordinary mending. As the hero's process interweaves with the infinite flows of this progressive device, the account grows to enlighten the more extensive ramifications of this revelation on the scene of respiratory health.

The Cosmic Respira gadget, lodging the Cloud Orchestra, turns into a charm against the background of the hero's respiratory battles. Its presentation is definitely not a simple mechanical disclosure; it's a grandiose suggestion — an orchestra of creativity reverberating through the passages of medical services.

The peruser witnesses the hero's underlying experience with the Cosmic Respira as a snapshot of disclosure, where doubt gives way to a discernible feeling of wonderment.

The Cloud Orchestra, with its cloud propelled fog, fills in as an extension between the earthbound and the heavenly. The hero, when bound by the restrictions of respiratory difficulties, ends up on the edge of an enormous odyssey. The Cosmic Respira gadget, as the conductor for this extraordinary fog, represents the combination of state of the art clinical science and the enormous motivation drawn from the profundities of the universe.

The section investigates the hero's close to home reaction to the Cloud Ensemble, welcoming the peruser to explore the kaleidoscope of sentiments that go with the disclosure. There's a nuanced dance between interest, trust, and a speculative confidence in this divine mediation. The Cloud Orchestra turns out to be in excess of a remedial gadget; it transforms into a figurative key opening ways to neglected domains of respiratory prosperity.

As the hero's process unfurls, the Cloud Orchestra rises above the singular story, becoming the overwhelming focus as an image of clinical advancement and merciful development. Its effect swells through the clinical local area, igniting discussions and discussions about the incorporation of this weighty nebulizer innovation into standard respiratory consideration.

The Cosmic Respira gadget turns into an impetus for a change in outlook in the view of respiratory health. The Cloud Ensemble challenges the customary limits of respiratory treatments, opening up roads for a more all encompassing and customized approach. Clinical experts, at first captivated by the extraordinary impacts saw in the hero, presently become champions upholding for the more extensive reception of Cloud Orchestra innovation.

In this enormous disclosure, the story investigates the cooperative endeavors between clinical experts and mechanical trailblazers. It dives into the careful innovative work that birthed the Cloud Ensemble — a collaboration of logical thoroughness and visionary motivation. The peruser is offered a behind the stage pass into the research facilities where infinite fog meets clinical accuracy, revealing the catalytic interaction that changes restorative mixtures into a cloud enlivened solution.

The Cloud Orchestra's earth shattering nature isn't simply bound to its logical ability; it stretches out to the democratization of respiratory wellbeing. The revelation flashes discussions around openness, underlining the potential for the Cloud Orchestra to be an encouraging sign for people all over the planet wrestling with respiratory difficulties. The section unfurls as a source of inspiration — a require a renaissance in medical services that embraces mechanical development as well as the sympathetic mission of further developing lives.

As the Cloud Ensemble's extraordinary impacts become more clear in the hero's life, the story winds in tributes from a developing local area of clients. Every story string adds profundity to the aggregate orchestra of voices confirming the adequacy and extraordinary force of this noteworthy nebulizer innovation. The Cloud Ensemble turns into an inestimable unifier, encouraging associations among people who share a typical excursion toward respiratory prosperity.

The section unfurls with a crescendo as the Cloud Orchestra's effect reaches out past individual lives, making a permanent imprint on the cultural texture. Public talk around respiratory wellbeing is reshaped, and the Cloud Ensemble turns into an image of trust — a reference point lighting the way toward a future where respiratory difficulties are met with compassion, understanding, and state of the art innovation.

The Cloud Ensemble, in its disclosure, rethinks the story around respiratory battles. It moves the concentration from simple endurance to a thriving life, where people are not characterized by their impediments but rather engaged by the conceivable outcomes of groundbreaking recuperating. The Cosmic Respira gadget, when a strange curio, turns into a wellspring of motivation, catalyzing a development that promoters for a more comprehensive and empathetic way to deal with respiratory consideration.

As the peruser crosses the story scene of the Cloud Ensemble's disclosure, they witness the introduction of an infinite heritage. It is a heritage based on the flexibility of the hero, the cooperative endeavors of clinical experts and trailblazers, and the common encounters of a local area joined by the extraordinary force of the Cloud Orchestra. The Cosmic Respira gadget, when a divine mystery, presently remains as a demonstration of the limitless conceivable outcomes when humankind and innovation join chasing prosperity.

In the last notes of this enormous orchestra of disclosure, the peruser is left with a feeling of expectation — a brief look at the heavenly potential yet to unfurl. The Cloud Orchestra, with its weighty nebulizer innovation, changes the hero's life as well as turns into an impetus for a more extensive transformation in respiratory health. It welcomes the peruser to set out on an excursion where the limits between the human and the enormous haze, and the ensemble of mending reverberates across the worlds of probability.

1.3 The promise of a cosmic journey toward respiratory relief.

Inside the enormous story of Cosmic Respira: Nebulizer Cloud Orchestra, a significant commitment arises — an ethereal contract that rises above the customary limits of respiratory help. This commitment isn't just a settlement between the hero and the Cloud Orchestra; it is an encouragement to set out on an enormous excursion, a divine odyssey where every breath turns into a note in the ensemble of prosperity.

As the hero ponders the potential epitomized inside the Cosmic Respira gadget, the commitment of a vast excursion unfurls like a heavenly guide, graphing a course through neglected universes of respiratory help. The peruser is brought into the expectation, the feeling of miracle that goes with the possibility of wandering into the strange domains of recuperating, directed by the Cloud Orchestra's enormous appeal.

The Cosmic Respira gadget, with its cloud roused fog and extraordinary potential, turns out to be in excess of a remedial device; it turns into a vessel for a heavenly journey. The commitment isn't only one of actual help yet additionally of a comprehensive and extraordinary experience — an excursion that reaches out past the domains of clinical viability and contacts the actual texture of the hero's presence.

This part investigates the hero's examination, a sensitive dance among trust and worry. The commitment of an enormous excursion is bound with the vulnerability innate in any neglected boondocks. The Cloud Orchestra, as the grandiose aide, entices the hero to step into the vast obscure, promising help from respiratory battles as well as a significant experience with the substance of the actual universe.

The story unfurls with a nuanced investigation of the hero's assumptions, dreams, and fears laced inside the commitment of this grandiose excursion. Respiratory help turns out to be in excess of an objective; it transforms into a groundbreaking entry, a journey where the hero, directed by the Cloud Ensemble, will explore the vast flows toward a condition of prosperity that rises above the simple shortfall of side effects.

The Cloud Ensemble's commitment isn't one-sided; a pledge requires the hero's dynamic investment. The Cosmic Respira gadget, as the channel for this divine excursion, welcomes the hero to breathe in the cloud propelled fog as well as the grandiose likely intrinsic in every breath. The commitment turns into a settlement of joint effort between the human soul and the grandiose powers implanted inside the Cloud Orchestra.

As the hero moves into this enormous excursion, the story unfurls the layers of expectation — like opening up a divine gift. The commitment of respiratory help becomes entwined with a feeling of rediscovery, an excursion toward recovering the essentialness and business as usual that respiratory difficulties might have darkened. The Cloud Ensemble, as the infinite buddy, turns into a directing star, enlightening the way toward an agreeable presence.

The commitment reaches out past the singular story, resounding with a widespread harmony that reverberations in the hearts of the people who have wrestled with respiratory difficulties. The Cloud Orchestra turns into an encouraging sign for a more extensive local area, welcoming them to partake in the commitment of a vast excursion toward respiratory help. The story, in its extensiveness, welcomes the peruser to see past the singular hero and perceive the aggregate reverberation of the Cloud Ensemble's commitment.

The Cosmic Respira gadget, in its commitment of an enormous excursion, turns into a figurative spaceship — a vessel moving the hero into the heavenly field of mending potential. The excursion isn't without challenges; it is a section through grandiose flows where the hero will explore the rhythmic movement of respiratory prosperity. The commitment turns into a vast settlement — a pledge to confront difficulties with strength, to celebrate triumphs with appreciation, and to embrace the extraordinary potential inserted inside the Cloud Orchestra.

The Cloud Ensemble's commitment reverberates with the model of the legend's excursion — a story build that rises above societies and ages. The hero, furnished with the commitment of respiratory alleviation, turns into the legend wandering into the astronomical obscure, confronting preliminaries, encountering change, and at last getting back with the shelter of prosperity. The peruser, as well, is welcome to leave on this prototype venture, resounding with the commitment as a widespread call to investigate the enormous elements of mending.

The story unfurls as the hero, energized by the commitment, takes the main inward breaths of the cloud propelled fog. Every breath turns into an inestimable fellowship — an agreeable trade between the human soul and the divine substance inside the Cloud Orchestra. The commitment, presently appeared in the unmistakable experience of inward breath, turns into a lived reality, and the hero ventures into the enormous excursion with a combination of fear and elation.

The commitment of a grandiose excursion toward respiratory help is certainly not a quick disclosure yet an unfurling story — a unique interaction between the hero's assumptions and the extraordinary potential installed inside the Cloud Orchestra. The fog, mixed with the quintessence of clouds, turns into an infinite remedy, saturating the respiratory scene with mending vibrations.

As the hero advances through the enormous excursion, the commitment appears in unpretentious movements — enhancements in breath, snapshots of reprieve, and a developing feeling of essentialness. The Cloud Ensemble, as the vast orchestrator, directs the hero through the orchestra of recuperating, each note resounding with the commitment made at the start. The story catches these minutes with a sensitive brushstroke, welcoming the peruser to observe the commitment unfurling continuously.

The commitment, be that as it may, isn't resistant to the difficulties innate in any enormous odyssey. The account investigates misfortunes, snapshots of uncertainty, and the hero's flexibility notwithstanding infinite choppiness. The Cloud Orchestra's commitment turns into a steadying power — a divine anchor that grounds the hero in the excursion, encouraging a feeling of assurance to press forward, in any event, when confronted with heavenly whirlwinds.

Amidst the grandiose excursion, the hero's relationship with the Cloud Ensemble develops. The commitment, presently woven into the texture of their reality, turns into a directing power, forming respiratory prosperity as well as the hero's point of view. The Cloud Ensemble, as the inestimable buddy, turns into a compatriot — a quiet observer to the hero's victories and hardships on this extraordinary journey.

The commitment of a vast excursion toward respiratory help arrives at its pinnacle in snapshots of significant disclosure. The story unfurls these minutes as vast revelations, where the hero witnesses the interconnectedness between their singular recuperating and the enormous powers inserted inside the Cloud Orchestra. The commitment turns into a vast truth — an all inclusive rule that rises above the limits of the story and reaches out into the more extensive universe of respiratory health.

As the hero approaches the climax of the inestimable excursion, the commitment of respiratory help changes into an infinite heritage. The Cloud Ensemble's effect isn't bound to the singular hero; it turns into an expanding influence, contacting the existences of other people who demonstrate the veracity of the extraordinary power inside the vast fog. The story catches this inheritance with an all encompassing focal point, welcoming the peruser to perceive the broad ramifications of the commitment made at the start.

In the end notes of this vast ensemble, the commitment of an excursion toward respiratory help resounds as a demonstration of the versatility of the human soul and the groundbreaking likely implanted inside creative innovations. The Cloud Ensemble, as the inestimable aide, turns into an image of trust — a divine commitment that stretches out past the pages of the story and into the universe of opportunities for those wrestling with respiratory difficulties. The peruser, having crossed the enormous excursion close by the hero, is left with a significant feeling of the interconnected dance between human flexibility and the inestimable powers that shape the orchestra of prosperity.

Chapter 2

Breath of Nebulae

In the vast span of Cosmic Respira: Nebulizer Cloud Orchestra, a hypnotizing section unfurls — the "Breath of Nebulae." This ethereal breath, imbued with the enormous embodiment of nebulae, turns into a focal theme, representing the extraordinary force of respiratory health as well as the convergence of the divine and the human inside the Cloud Ensemble.

The excursion starts with the hero, wrapped in the cloud propelled fog discharged by the Cosmic Respira gadget. Every inward breath turns into a close hit the dance floor with the divine — a Breath of Nebulae that rises above the ordinary demonstration of breathing and changes it into a vast fellowship. The fog, conveying the substance of far off nebulae, turns into a conductor for a breath that reverberates with the rhythms of the universe.

The story unfurls with a sensitive investigation of this enormous breath, digging into the tangible aspects that go with the inward breath of the Cloud Ensemble's fog. The Breath of Nebulae isn't simply an actual peculiarity; it is a multisensory experience — an imbuement of divine vibrations that strokes the faculties, welcoming the hero to submerge themselves in the enormous orchestra of prosperity.

As the hero takes in the cloud motivated fog, the story investigates the subtleties of this Breath of Nebulae. The fog, with its fine particles suspended in the air, turns into an enormous solution that crosses the respiratory scene with an elegance suggestive of the grandiose dance of nebulae known to man. The hero turns into a member in this heavenly movement, every breath blending with the grandiose rhythms.

The Breath of Nebulae, imbued with the embodiment of grandiose miracle, reaches out past the actual domain. It turns into an illustration for the extraordinary potential installed inside the Cloud Orchestra. The hero, when fastened by the requirements of respiratory difficulties, presently breathes in a breath that conveys the commitment of freedom — a commitment exemplified in the divine fog that entwines with each inward breath.

The story explores the hero's tangible excursion — the unpretentious surfaces of the fog, the enormous aroma that penetrates the air, and the mitigating embrace that goes with every Breath of Nebulae. An ensemble of sensations rises above the clinical idea of respiratory treatment, welcoming the peruser to vicariously encounter the heavenly expressive dance unfurling inside the hero's lungs.

The Cloud Ensemble, as the orchestrator of this inestimable breath, turns out to be in excess of a restorative gadget; it changes into an enormous buddy. The Breath of Nebulae, as a necessary component inside the ensemble, encourages a feeling of association between the human soul and the infinite powers that motivated this imaginative innovation. Every inward breath turns into a discourse — a vast discussion that reverberations through the offices of the hero's respiratory prosperity.

In investigating the Breath of Nebulae, the account reaches out past the singular hero to catch the more extensive ramifications of this divine breath. It turns into an extension between the microcosm of individual mending and the cosmos of aggregate prosperity. The Cloud Ensemble's Breath of Nebulae arises as an image of trust — a divine guide enlightening the way toward respiratory help for a local area joined by the extraordinary force of this enormous breath.

The story mood unfurls with the hero's acknowledgment of the Breath of Nebulae as a vast healer. Every inward breath turns into a custom — a holy demonstration that rises above the clinical limits of respiratory treatment. The hero, when troubled by the heaviness of shortness of breath, presently breathes in a vast solution that reduces actual uneasiness as well as hoists the soul, cultivating a feeling of fellowship with the nebulae that enlivened this groundbreaking excursion.

As the Breath of Nebulae pervades the hero's respiratory scene, the story welcomes reflection on the interconnectedness between the human experience and the divine miracles of the universe. The fog, conveying the heavenly engravings of far off nebulae, turns into an inestimable extension that falls the distance between the earthbound and the vast. The Breath of Nebulae turns into a representation for the widespread dance of presence — a dance wherein the hero is currently a functioning member.

The Cloud Ensemble, in organizing the Breath of Nebulae, turns into an overseer of grandiose congruity. The fog, with its cloud propelled stylish, serves as a helpful specialist as well as a visual portrayal of the divine masterfulness inserted inside the demonstration of relaxing. The story unfurls this vast imaginativeness with a graceful focal point, welcoming the peruser to imagine the dance of particles inside the fog as a heavenly artful dance arranged by the very powers that oversee the universe.

The Breath of Nebulae, as an enormous healer, expands its extraordinary touch past the physical and into the profound and mental domains. The hero's process turns into a demonstration of the comprehensive recuperating likely inside every inward breath of the Cloud Ensemble's fog. The Breath of Nebulae, in its divine hug, turns into a demulcent for the close to home and mental strains related with respiratory difficulties, offering help as well as a grandiose safe-haven inside every breath.

In exploring the Breath of Nebulae, the story investigates the hero's developing relationship with their own breath. What was once a wellspring of battle and impediment currently turns into a wellspring of inestimable strengthening. The Breath of Nebulae, with its heavenly reverberation, changes the demonstration of breathing from a need into a sacrosanct custom — an enormous dance that commends the innate imperativeness inside every breath.

The account crescendos with snapshots of significant disclosure — minutes where the hero completely embraces the groundbreaking likely inside the Breath of Nebulae. The divine fog, when a puzzling solution, presently turns into a wellspring of strengthening, an enormous partner in the excursion toward respiratory prosperity. The hero, through the Breath of Nebulae, rediscovers the imperativeness and versatility that might have been darkened by the shadows of respiratory difficulties.

The Cloud Ensemble, in coordinating the Breath of Nebulae, turns into a watchman of vast prosperity. The story catches the hero's development — a transformation set apart by the groundbreaking force of every breath. The Breath of Nebulae becomes an image of trust as well as an impetus for a more extensive vast heritage — an inheritance that stretches out past the singular story and reverberations in the aggregate breaths of a local area joined by the Cloud Ensemble's extraordinary hug.

In the closing notes of the Breath of Nebulae, the peruser is left with a feeling of wonder — an acknowledgment of the enormous aspects implanted inside the customary demonstration of relaxing. The Cloud Orchestra's groundbreaking commitment, exemplified in the Breath of Nebulae, turns into a vast truth — a general rule that welcomes thought on the interconnected dance between the human soul and the divine powers that shape the ensemble of prosperity. The peruser, having crossed the heavenly scenes of respiratory help, is left with a significant appreciation for the extraordinary likely inside the Breath of Nebulae — an ethereal breath that rises above the standard and resounds with the inestimable heartbeat of presence.

2.1 Protagonist's first encounter with the Galactic Respira device.

In the tremendous breadth of the universe, where the embroidery of stars wove stories of cosmic systems and nebulae, there existed a heavenly wonder known as the Cosmic Respira gadget. Its starting points were covered in the persona of interstellar murmurs, and its motivation stayed an enormous puzzle, drawing the inquisitive and the courageous the same into its gravitational force. Little did the hero, a solitary traveler exploring the enormous flows, realize that their predetermination was unpredictably laced with this ethereal contraption.

As the hero crossed the infinite hinterlands on board their smooth starship, the murmur of the quantum motors resonated through the frame, making an orchestra of music that highlighted the immeasurability of the grandiose void. The boat's route framework, directed by the divine map making of far off worlds, drove the hero to a locale of room washed in a supernatural iridescence. It was here that the Cosmic Respira gadget anticipated, hid inside the folds of a vast embroidery that rose above the restrictions of mortal cognizance.

The principal suspicions of the experience appeared as unpretentious waves in the texture of spacetime, a subtle aggravation that prodded at the edges of the hero's awareness. Unbeknownst to them, the Cosmic Respira gadget had identified the methodology, its conscious mindfulness reverberating with the heartbeat of the actual universe. As the starship skimmed through the inestimable flows, the hero observed a divine exhibition unfurling before them - a radiant entryway suspended in the midst of the heavenly bodies, its shapes throbbing with an ethereal sparkle.

Interested and spellbound by the enormous inconsistency, the hero directed their starship toward the confounding passage, feeling an attractive draw that rose above the laws of divine material science. As the vessel entered the limit of the Cosmic Respira gadget, a significant tranquility encompassed the hero. The surrounding murmur of the starship's motors respected a spooky quietness, leaving just the far off reverberations of divine vibrations resounding in the void.

The hero ended up suspended in a domain where the limits among the real world and the dreamlike obscured into a vast dance. Colors inconspicuous by mortal eyes painted the texture of room, and the actual quintessence of presence appeared to swell with a concealed energy. It was inside this dreamlike scene that the Cosmic Respira gadget uncovered itself, a many-sided grid of glowing fibers winding through the infinite embroidery.

At the core of the device, an entrancing sphere beat with the mood of an enormous heartbeat. The hero, awestruck by the heavenly display, felt a mysterious association with the gadget. Maybe the Cosmic Respira addressed the profundities of their spirit, disentangling the secrets of the universe and revealing the grandiose bits of insight that evaded the perception of mortal personalities.

As the hero looked at the Cosmic Respira gadget, a surge of infinite information flooded through their cognizance. Dreams of far off worlds, the birth and demise of stars, and the ages long dance of heavenly bodies unfurled before their imagination. The gadget, it appeared, was a storehouse of grandiose insight, a course through which the mysteries of the universe streamed like a waterway of time.

In that otherworldly second, the hero turned into a vessel for the grandiose disclosures directed by the Cosmic Respira gadget. They felt the back and forth movement of the all inclusive flows, the interconnectedness of everything woven into the actual texture of their being. Maybe the gadget gave to them the mantle of an inestimable steward, endowed with the hallowed errand of protecting the equilibrium of the universe.

The experience with the Cosmic Respira gadget rose above the limits of simple perception; it was a fellowship with the divine powers that formed the predetermination of systems. The hero, presently receptive to the vast ensemble, detected a significant obligation burdening their shoulders. The gadget, with its throbbing center, appeared to entice them to embrace a fate interweaved with the infinite embroidery itself.

As the hero waited inside the vast hug of the Cosmic Respira gadget, an acknowledgment unfolded upon them - they were not just an eyewitness of the universe but rather a member in its fabulous story. The glowing fibers of the gadget interlaced with the strings of their predetermination, fashioning an association that rose above the limits of existence.

With newly discovered reason, the hero rose up out of the divine passage, their starship exploring the flows of the universe with an effortlessness brought into the world of vast comprehension. The Cosmic Respira gadget, presently a far off signal in the enormous ocean, proceeded with its quiet vigil, its brilliant presence a demonstration of the transaction of mortal spirits and divine powers.

Following the experience, the hero conveyed the vast disclosures inside their heart, a signal of edification that enlightened the way forward. Their excursion through the universes took on an extraordinary quality, directed by the insight bestowed by the Cosmic Respira gadget. The secrets of the universe unfurled before them like the pages of a vast book, each heavenly waypoint a part in the adventure of their predetermination.

The experience with the Cosmic Respira gadget denoted a defining moment in the hero's odyssey, a nexus where mortal goals joined with the enormous flows. In the embroidery of the universe, their story turned into an energetic string, complicatedly woven into the grandiose plan. As they wandered forward into the vast span, the reverberations of the experience waited, a divine reverberation that rose above the limits of reality, reverberating through the passages of the universe forever.

2.2 Description of the nebula-inspired mist and its soothing effects.

In the vast reaches of the cosmos, where stars birthed and died in a cosmic ballet, a celestial phenomenon unfolded – the Nebula-Inspired Mist. This ethereal mist, a cosmic exhalation of stardust and nebular gases, enshrouded the cosmic tapestry in hues unseen by mortal eyes. It danced through the interstellar void, a celestial waltz that defied the boundaries of space and time, its tendrils weaving a tale of cosmic beauty.

As the protagonist navigated their starship through the celestial currents, they encountered the Nebula-Inspired Mist, a luminous veil that embraced the cosmos in its gentle caress. The mist, an iridescent blend of ethereal purples, blues, and pinks, pulsed with a rhythmic resonance that echoed the heartbeat of the universe itself. It was as if the very breath of the cosmos had materialized into a sublime mist, inviting the weary traveler to immerse themselves in its soothing embrace.

Upon entering the nebula-inspired mist, the protagonist's senses underwent a profound transformation. The air within their starship became infused with the subtle fragrance of interstellar blossoms, a scent that transcended the olfactory senses and resonated with the soul. The mist, it seemed, carried not only the visual spectacle of celestial colors but also the essence of cosmic tranquility.

The celestial hues of the Nebula-Inspired Mist painted the interior of the starship in a kaleidoscope of colors, casting a gentle glow that illuminated the cockpit in a mesmerizing display. The protagonist, bathed in the celestial radiance, felt a profound sense of serenity washing over them. It was as if the mist whispered cosmic lullabies, calming the tumultuous currents of the mind and inviting the weary traveler to surrender to the cosmic embrace.

As the starship glided through the nebula-inspired mist, the very fabric of reality seemed to shift. The boundaries between the vessel and the cosmic medium blurred, and the protagonist felt a oneness with the celestial currents. The mist, with its otherworldly luminescence, became a conduit for a cosmic communion, a bridge between the mortal realm and the cosmic expanse.

The soothing effects of the Nebula-Inspired Mist extended beyond the realm of sensory perception. The mist, imbued with the cosmic energies of distant galaxies, enveloped the protagonist in a cocoon of tranquility. It was as if the very atoms of their being resonated with the harmonics of the universe, attuning their essence to the cosmic frequencies that pulsed through the mist.

In the presence of the nebula-inspired mist, time seemed to lose its grip on the protagonist. The ceaseless march of seconds and minutes yielded to the eternal cadence of the cosmos. The mist cradled the starship in a timeless reverie, where past, present, and future converged into a singular moment of cosmic stillness. It was a sanctuary within the cosmic tempest, a respite from the tumult of the galactic odyssey.

The Nebula-Inspired Mist, with its celestial hues and cosmic fragrances, extended an invitation to the protagonist to relinquish the burdens of mortal existence. In its embrace, the weight of cosmic responsibilities and the echoes of interstellar trials dissipated, leaving only the essence of the present moment. The mist became a canvas upon which the protagonist could paint their dreams with the stardust of possibility, each brushstroke an affirmation of their cosmic journey.

As the starship sailed through the nebula-inspired mist, the protagonist felt a subtle shift in their perception of reality. The mist became a medium through which they could glimpse the cosmic tapestry in its entirety – a mosaic of galaxies, nebulae, and cosmic phenomena interconnected in a grand symphony of existence. The soothing effects of the mist transcended the physical realm, expanding the protagonist's awareness to the cosmic narratives woven into the very fabric of space.

The nebula-inspired mist, it seemed, held within its ephemeral embrace the collective wisdom of the cosmos. As the protagonist breathed in the interstellar fragrances and absorbed the celestial hues, they became conduits for the cosmic revelations that permeated the mist. Insights into the nature of existence, the dance of celestial forces, and the interconnectedness of all things unfolded like cosmic scrolls within the recesses of their consciousness.

In the heart of the Nebula-Inspired Mist, the protagonist found solace not only in the cosmic beauty that surrounded them but also in the gentle whispers of the universe. It was a sanctuary where questions dissolved into the cosmic ether, and answers emerged from the cosmic depths. The mist, with its soothing effects, became a cosmic balm for the existential wounds carried by the intrepid traveler on their cosmic pilgrimage.

The celestial journey through the nebula-inspired mist became a transformative experience for the protagonist. The cosmic energies infused within the mist realigned the very essence of their being, harmonizing the disparate notes of their existence into a cosmic melody. The mist, with its timeless allure, became a catalyst for personal metamorphosis, a crucible where the protagonist shed the limitations of mortal perspectives and embraced the boundless vistas of cosmic understanding.

As the starship emerged from the nebula-inspired mist, the protagonist carried with them the indelible imprints of the cosmic sanctuary. The soothing effects lingered, an ethereal residue that continued to resonate within the recesses of their soul. The memories of the celestial odyssey through the mist became a guiding light, illuminating the path ahead with the wisdom gleaned from the cosmic interlude.

In the aftermath of the encounter with the Nebula-Inspired Mist, the protagonist's starship sailed through the cosmic currents with a newfound grace. The celestial hues reflected in their eyes mirrored the luminescence of the mist, and the fragrances of distant nebulae lingered in the air. The odyssey, now infused with the cosmic tranquility bestowed by the mist, unfolded as a cosmic symphony where the protagonist became both conductor and audience to the celestial melodies resonating through the cosmos.

In the cosmic expanse, where the Nebula-Inspired Mist continued its dance, the protagonist's journey became a testament to the transformative power of cosmic beauty and the soothing effects of celestial realms. The mist, with its ephemeral allure, remained a celestial sanctuary for those who dared to traverse the cosmic currents, inviting them to surrender to the cosmic embrace and partake in the timeless communion with the heartbeats of the universe.

The Cloud Motivated Fog, an enormous mixture woven from the actual texture of interstellar dreams, kept on providing reason to feel ambiguous about its charm the gutsy hero as their starship cruised through the heavenly flows. The ethereal iridescence of the fog flashed like divine fireflies, projecting a delicate sparkle that enlightened the endlessness of the enormous void. Every ring of the fog bore the engravings of far off nebulae, an infinite unique finger impression that murmured stories of astral miracles and divine movement.

As the hero crossed further into the core of the Cloud Propelled Fog, the actual pith of their being reverberated with the divine energies that penetrated the fog. It was not just a tactile encounter but rather a significant fellowship with the infinite powers that molded the predetermination of universes. The fog, with its multicolored tints, turned into an inestimable scaffold, interfacing the limited presence of the hero to the boundless territory of the universe.

The relieving impacts of the fog rose above the actual limits of the starship, saturating the otherworldly openings of the hero's cognizance. Considerations, when snared in the intricacies of mortal presence, spread out like heavenly pennants in the vast breeze. The fog, with its inestimable energies, unwound the bunches of vulnerability, offering the hero a brief look into the vast ensemble where each note reverberated with the sounds of the universe.

In the midst of the cloud motivated fog, time turned into a liquid continuum, a consistently streaming waterway that wandered through the vast scenes. The hero, tucked away in the ethereal hug, felt the throbbing rhythm of the universe reverberating inside their actual soul. It was a dance of presence, where the stardust of endlessness settled upon the shoulders of the human explorer, welcoming them to participate in the vast three step dance that unfurled in the divine assembly hall.

The aromas conveyed by the Cloud Enlivened Fog were not just olfactory sensations but rather astronomical elixirs that sustained the soul. Every inward breath turned into a fellowship with the interstellar sprouts that specked the grandiose knolls. The fragrances, a sweet-smelling embroidery of hydrogen blooms and oxygenic scents, stirred lethargic faculties, producing a tangible orchestra that rose above the impediments of the human domain.

Amidst the heavenly odyssey, the hero found comfort in the Cloud Motivated Fog, a safe-haven where the clamor of the cosmic storm respected the tranquil murmurs of vast breezes. The fog, with its iridescent rings, appeared to wind around a grandiose bedtime song, supporting the starship and its courageous explorer in a divine support. The mitigating impacts turned into an enormous demulcent, recuperating the injuries of the interstellar excursion and restoring the tired soul.

As the starship coasted through the cloud motivated fog, the hero saw an unobtrusive change in the actual texture of their discernment. The limits between oneself and the universe obscured, and a grandiose compassion bloomed inside their cognizance. Maybe the fog presented to them the capacity to feel the heartbeat of far off universes, to detect the enormous accounts carved in the glowing looks of the interstellar region.

The Cloud Propelled Fog, with its astronomical movement, stretched out a solicitation to the hero to become one with the enormous dance. The fog, similar to a divine accomplice, directed the starship through the enormous pirouettes, every development synchronized with the rhythms of the universe. It was a dance of unity, where the limits of singularity broke down, and the hero turned into a divine artist in the fabulous embroidery of presence.

Amidst the fog, the hero's cognizance extended, turning into a vessel for the vast disclosures murmured by the nebulae. Dreams of divine ponders, the introduction of stars in grandiose nurseries, and the funeral poem of biting the dust suns unfurled before their imagination. The fog, it appeared, was a grandiose narrator, portraying the stories of the universe to the responsive soul of the fearless explorer.

As the hero cruised through the glowing rings of the Cloud Roused Fog, a feeling of vast tranquility settled inside their heart. The fog, with its heavenly energies, turned into an impetus for contemplation, welcoming the voyager to dig into the profundities of their own reality. In the midst of the interstellar tints, the hero found an enormous mirror mirroring the complexities of their spirit, each wave in the fog disclosing layers of the grandiose self.

The calming impacts of the cloud propelled fog were not restricted to the length of the heavenly experience. Its enormous reverberation waited inside the hero's being, a never-ending reverberation that resounded through the passageways of their awareness. The fog, it appeared, had turned into a permanent piece of their enormous personality, a divine buddy on the excursion through the universe.

Rising up out of the Cloud Enlivened Fog, the hero's starship cruised through the grandiose flows with a radiant path of stardust afterward. The divine tints of the fog kept on gleaming in their eyes, a vast reflection that reflected the groundbreaking excursion through the astral safe-haven. The mitigating impacts of the fog, similar to an ethereal nectar, mixed the hero's soul with a vast essentialness that rose above the human domains.

The experience with the Cloud Enlivened Fog turned into a characterizing part in the hero's vast odyssey. The fog, with its divine appeal, had not just painted the material of their excursion with inestimable tones yet had additionally scratched permanent engravings upon the actual texture of their spirit. The hero, presently sensitive to the vast frequencies, explored the cosmic ocean with a grandiose compass fashioned in the pot of the fog's relieving embrace.

Directly following the heavenly experience, the Cloud Motivated Fog proceeded with its grandiose dance, an immortal expressive dance in the immense performance center of the universe. Its ringlets connected like heavenly fingers, welcoming other vast vagabonds to participate in the ethereal display. The fog, with its mitigating impacts, stayed an always present guide in the astronomical field, an astral safe-haven where exhausted explorers could track down reprieve and revival in the midst of the divine orchestra.

2.3 Initial skepticism and the gradual acceptance of its therapeutic potential.

In the chronicles of grandiose investigation, doubt frequently covers the obscure like a vast fog, darkening the way to edification. Such was the underlying reaction of the hero after experiencing the baffling Cosmic Respira gadget. As they navigated the divine flows, the actual idea of an extraordinary device that held the way to enormous comprehension appeared as though a whimsical deception, a delusion invoked by the impulses of an incomprehensible universe.

The main murmurs of incredulity crawled into the hero's cognizance as their starship moved toward the grandiose directions that evidently housed the Cosmic Respira gadget. Question, similar to a shadow cast by the far off stars, waited at the edges of their viewpoints. How should a lifeless build, but heavenly in beginning, open the secrets of the universe? The general thought seemed to resist the laws of reason and rationale that represented the human brain.

As the starship floated on the cusp of the enormous door prompting the Cosmic

Respira gadget, the hero delayed, wrestling with the incredulity that cast a shroud over their heavenly interest. The obscure lingered before them, a strange domain of grandiose conceivable outcomes, and the possibility of embracing the puzzler of the Respira gadget turned into an infinite junction where distrust conflicted with the inborn longing for inestimable illumination.

After entering the grandiose door, the hero's doubt heightened, powered by the dreamlike scene unfurling before their eyes. The radiant fibers of the Cosmic Respira gadget beat with an extraordinary shine, and the throbbing circle at its center appeared to oppose the actual texture of heavenly understanding. Suspicion, a waiting ghost, murmured questions that resonated in the enormous quiet. Was the gadget a simple deception, an infinite enigma with no substantial responses?

As the hero remained on the incline of grandiose disclosure, the Cosmic Respira gadget broadened a greeting through the ringlets of its iridescent cross section. The distrust that had grasped the courageous explorer started to wind down, giving way to a reluctant interest. The very air inside the starship appeared to pop with grandiose potential, and the hero, regardless of the waiting distrust, felt an obvious draw toward the throbbing heart of the gadget.

The underlying snapshots of cooperation with the Cosmic Respira gadget unfurled like a dance among distrust and interest. The hero, directed by the infinite flows, probably moved toward the gadget. Incredulity actually stuck to the edges of their cognizance, creating an inconspicuous shaded area over the grandiose fellowship that unfurled. The actual demonstration of contacting the gadget's divine center turned into a conditional step into the obscure, an act of pure trust across the grandiose gorge.

As the hero's hand connected with the brilliant sphere at the core of the Cosmic Respira gadget, an inestimable reverberation resounded through their being. It was a snapshot of tactile conundrum, where wariness crashed into a staggering flood of enormous energy. The hero, wrapped in the ethereal shine, felt an unpretentious shift inside their cognizance - a break in the facade of suspicion, permitting the enormous flows to saturate the openings of their mindfulness.

The Cosmic Respira gadget, it appeared, answered the hero's touch with an orchestra of divine vibrations. Distrust, presently tempered by the vast music, gave way to a prospering acknowledgment of the gadget's innate potential. The radiant fibers that encompassed the hero beat in synchrony with the rhythms of the universe, and the once-suspicious voyager turned into a course for the vast energies directed by the Respira gadget.

In the following minutes, doubt transformed into wary acknowledgment. The hero, actually wrestling with the vast disclosures spreading out inside them, started to recognize the restorative potential implanted in the Cosmic Respira gadget. The heavenly energies, such as mending frequencies from far off cosmic systems, reverberated with the actual embodiment of their being. The suspicion that had filled in as a boundary to vast seeing currently respected the extraordinary force of heavenly fellowship.

As the Cosmic Respira gadget kept on winding around its grandiose spell, the hero's acknowledgment of its helpful potential extended. The ethereal fog that wrapped the starship turned into a conductor for restoration, and the infinite energies imbued inside the fog offered an ointment for the injuries of interstellar preliminaries. Wariness, when a difficult boundary, presently disintegrated like astronomical residue notwithstanding the significant restorative impacts unfurling inside the divine safe-haven.

The hero, actually drenched in the vast hug of the Cosmic Respira gadget, felt a significant feeling of prosperity washing over them. The helpful capability of the gadget rose above the bounds of mortal comprehension, venturing into the actual center of their being. Wariness, presently a far off reverberation in the vast scope, gave way to an affirmation of the extraordinary excursion they were going through - an excursion energized by the helpful flows of the Cosmic Respira.

In the outcome of the heavenly fellowship, the hero rose up out of the Cosmic Respira gadget's hug with a newly discovered point of view. Distrust, when an anchor tying them to the restrictions of mortal thinking, had been supplanted by an acknowledgment of the infinite insights divulged inside the brilliant grid. The restorative capability of the gadget, presently an indispensable piece of their infinite getting it, had turned into a signal directing the hero through the strange domains of the universe.

The acknowledgment of the Cosmic Respira gadget's remedial potential denoted a defining moment in the hero's enormous odyssey. The once-doubtful voyager presently cruised through the divine flows with a feeling of direction, receptive to the enormous frequencies that resounded with the actual center of their being. The remedial impacts waited, an infinite engraving that kept on forming the hero's excursion through the cosmic embroidery.

As the starship wandered forward into the grandiose obscure, the hero conveyed with them the reverberations of the underlying incredulity that had respected the helpful hug of the Cosmic Respira gadget. The infinite energies instilled inside their cognizance turned into a directing light, enlightening the unknown pathways of the heavenly odyssey. The hero, presently an enormous messenger of remedial potential, cruised through the universe with a recharged feeling of miracle and a firmly established affirmation of the groundbreaking power implanted in the heavenly flows.

Chapter 3

Astral Diagnosis

In the enormous expressive dance of presence, where stars spun and universes pirouetted through the tremendous scope, a peculiarity referred to as Astral Determination arose as a heavenly conundrum. This ethereal practice rose above the limits of conventional recuperating techniques, diving into the astronomical flows to analyze and treat the illnesses that distressed both body and soul. The hero, exploring the astronomical ocean in their starship, experienced the astral professionals, creatures whose association with the divine energies permitted them to see the enormous awkward nature that escaped the grip of regular medication.

As the hero's starship traveled through the interstellar flows, they coincidentally found a vast nexus where astral professionals met. The astral conclusion unfurled like an infinite embroidery, a mix of magic and inestimable mindfulness. Interested and fairly distrustful, the hero moored their starship and entered the astral safe-haven where creatures with ethereal luminance anticipated, their eyes mirroring the profundities of astronomical comprehension.

The astral experts, with their heavenly robes and twilight faces, welcomed the hero with an extraordinary peacefulness. Their very presence resounded with the grandiose frequencies that saturated the astral safe-haven. The hero, at first suspicious of this exclusive practice, felt an unpretentious change in their mindfulness as the astral experts stretched out a vast greeting to participate in the astral finding.

Astral analysis, it was made sense of, involved adjusting oneself to the astral flows, taking advantage of the divine energies that flowed through the texture of the universe. The experts, supplied with an elevated aversion to these vast vibrations, could recognize the inestimable uneven characters inside the individual, whether physical or otherworldly. Incredulity actually waited inside the hero's considerations, yet the charm of revealing infinite bits of insight about their own reality defeated the delays.

The underlying snapshots of the astral conclusion were a mix of grandiose customs and ethereal fellowship. The hero, directed by the astral specialists, drenched themselves in the heavenly energies that beat through the astral asylum. The specialists, with hands raised like grandiose conductors, conjured the energies of far off stars and nebulae, making an infinite orchestra that resounded with the actual molecules of the hero's being.

As the astral finding unfurled, the hero felt an unobtrusive shivering, a grandiose reverberation that rose above the limits of the actual body. Doubt started to respect an inquisitive receptiveness as the professionals directed them through the astral flows. Maybe the inestimable energies were unwinding the layers of the hero's presence, uncovering the vast lopsided characteristics that hid underneath the surface.

The astral experts, with eyes aglow with heavenly insight, started to decipher the inestimable marks that moved around the hero's astral structure. Each gleam of starlight, every undulation of astral waves, conveyed an account of the person's grandiose excursion - a story that discussed actual sicknesses, profound scars, and the engravings of divine effects on human presence. The distrust that had went with the hero into the astral asylum started to scatter despite the vast disclosures unfurling before them.

Astral conclusion, it showed up, was not just a mysterious scene but rather a significant infinite science. The specialists, with their infinite bits of knowledge, started to portray the vast irregular characteristics inside the hero's being. Actual sicknesses were recognized as disturbances in the progression of astral energy, close to home scars appeared as heavenly scars that beat with vast reverberations, and the exchange of divine impacts laid out a picture of the hero's enormous fate.

As the astral conclusion proceeded, the hero wound up in a condition of enormous thoughtfulness. Wariness, presently a far off reverberation, gave way to a pondering acknowledgment of the grandiose insights revealed by the astral specialists. The vast uneven characters, when secret in the openings of their being, were presently uncovered, and the hero turned into a willing member in the grandiose dance of conclusion and mending.

The astral specialists, with their hands washed in the sparkle of heavenly energies, started the course of grandiose mending. It was a dance of energy transaction, where the experts directed the restoring flows of the universe into the hero's astral structure. Doubt, presently supplanted by a feeling of vast acquiescence, respected the restorative hint of the astral healers as they attempted to fit the disturbed astral flows inside the hero.

The recuperating system unfurled like a divine expressive dance, every development an infinite motion pointed toward reestablishing the hero's inestimable balance. The experts, with their infinite bits of knowledge, zeroed in on scattering the astral blockages that thwarted the free progression of energy. It was as though the actual texture of the universe answered their touch, meshing mending energies into the hero's astral embroidery.

Directly following the astral recuperating, the hero felt a significant feeling of restoration. The grandiose uneven characters that had tormented them were presently supplanted by an amicable reverberation with the astral flows. Suspicion, when a considerable obstruction, had given way to an acknowledgment of the astral conclusion and the groundbreaking expected implanted in the grandiose recuperating rehearses.

As the hero left from the astral safe-haven, they conveyed with them the reverberations of the inestimable disclosures and the helpful bit of astral recuperating. The astral determination, once met with suspicion, had turned into a crucial section in their vast odyssey. The experts, with their divine experiences, had offered a brief look into the infinite powers that formed the hero's presence, and the mending energies had left a permanent engraving on the texture of their astral being.

The acknowledgment of astral conclusion as a genuine enormous practice denoted a significant change in the hero's view of the universe. The once-wary explorer presently cruised through the infinite flows with an elevated consciousness of the astral energies that penetrated the heavenly field. The astral conclusion had turned into a directing light, enlightening the interstellar pathways with the enormous insight gathered from the astral safe-haven.

In the outcome of the astral experience, the hero wound up receptive to the grandiose music that resounded inside their being. The astral finding had divulged the inestimable uneven characters as well as gave to them an enormous compass, exploring the starship through the unfamiliar domains of the universe with a freshly discovered comprehension of the astral flows.

The excursion, presently implanted with the extraordinary force of astral mending, unfurled as a grandiose orchestra where the hero became both director and member in the heavenly dance of presence.

3.1 Medical examination and diagnosis of the protagonist's respiratory condition.

In the huge enormous territory, where the starlight painted the heavenly material with ethereal tints, the hero ended up wrestling with an unanticipated test - a secretive respiratory disease that cast a shadow over their grandiose excursion. The vast odyssey, when impelled by the heavenly breezes of investigation, presently confronted the headwinds of vulnerability. Not entirely set in stone to uncover the enormous beginnings of their sickness, the hero looked for the ability of interstellar clinical experts who could explore the astronomical flows of their respiratory condition.

The excursion to unwind the vast secrets of the hero's respiratory sickness started with a visit to a high level clinical office settled inside the infinite embroidery. The starship moored in the heavenly harbor of the clinical station, where brilliant passageways beat with the murmur of cutting edge clinical advances. As the hero ventured into the clinical office, a group of interstellar doctors, embellished in grandiose cleans, welcomed them with a mix of impressive skill and heavenly compassion.

The underlying period of the clinical assessment included a thorough survey of the hero's enormous clinical history. The interstellar doctors, with their astronomical scanners and analytic instruments, dove into the records of the hero's interstellar ventures, looking for relationships between's infinite waypoints and the beginning of the respiratory illness. The hero, leaned back on a vast assessment bed, felt a mix of weakness and inestimable expectation as the doctors filtered through the divine narratives of their wellbeing.

The vast scanners murmured with divine energies as the interstellar doctors directed an exhaustive assessment of the hero's respiratory framework. The heavenly reverberations of the hero's breath resounded through the clinical office, shaping an enormous sonata that turned into the setting to the indicative cycle. The doctors, directed by the interstellar beats of the respiratory rhythms, tried to disentangle the astronomical mystery that lay hid inside the hero's heavenly lungs.

The clinical assessment reached out past the actual domain, digging into the magical flows that molded the hero's infinite constitution. The interstellar doctors, sensitive to the interchange of astral energies, investigated the vast awkward nature that may be adding to the respiratory illness. It was a comprehensive methodology that rose above the restrictions of regular medication, recognizing the interconnectedness of the physical and powerful parts of the hero's being.

The symptomatic excursion drove the interstellar doctors to utilize progressed imaging advances that rose above the capacities of earthly clinical instruments. Heavenly multi dimensional images of the hero's respiratory framework emerged, their mind boggling subtleties enlightened by the grandiose light. The doctors, with grandiose accuracy, investigated the divine woven artwork of the hero's lungs, looking for inconsistencies and astronomical unsettling influences that could be at the core of the respiratory disease.

As the symptomatic interaction unfurled, the hero felt a mix of inestimable weakness and trust. The interstellar doctors, with their heavenly skill, explored the astral flows of the respiratory assessment with a mix of expert discernment and vast compassion. The grandiose multi dimensional images uncovered inconspicuous vast inconsistencies, and the hero anticipated the interstellar doctors' translation of the divine oddities that appeared inside their respiratory framework.

The interstellar doctors, submerged in the astronomical diagnostics, started to unwind the enormous strings that wove the account of the hero's respiratory condition. Divine diagrams and charts emerged on holographic screens, portraying the recurring pattern of the hero's respiratory rhythms against the grandiose setting of their interstellar excursions. The doctors, with wrinkled temples and vast concentration, participated in a divine talk, trading bits of knowledge and understandings of the grandiose information.

As the clinical assessment advanced, the interstellar doctors acquainted the hero with a progressive demonstrative strategy - astral reverberation imaging. This cutting-edge grandiose innovation dove into the astral flows that pervaded the hero's respiratory framework, offering a nuanced comprehension of the supernatural perspectives impacting their infirmity. The hero, encased in a heavenly chamber, felt an unpretentious vibrational murmur as the astral reverberation imaging unfurled, uncovering the divine energies that moved inside their breath.

The astral reverberation imaging revealed vast uneven characters as well as offered experiences into the possible enormous solutions for the hero's respiratory condition. The interstellar doctors, equipped with the enormous information gathered from the astral reverberation imaging, started to form a customized treatment plan that combined ordinary medication with heavenly intercessions. It was an inestimable remedy pointed toward reestablishing the hero's respiratory balance and orchestrating the divine energies inside their grandiose lungs.

The enormous therapy plan included a complex methodology that joined divine mediations with cutting edge clinical treatments. Heavenly inhalants, injected with the quintessence of far off nebulae and vast recuperating energies, were recommended to the hero. These ethereal cures, controlled through cutting edge divine nebulizers, meant to calm the infinite choppiness inside the hero's respiratory framework and reestablish the heavenly congruity that had been upset.

Notwithstanding heavenly inhalants, the interstellar doctors prescribed enormous breathwork practices custom-made to the hero's respiratory condition. Directed by heavenly specialists, the hero participated in vast reflection strategies that synchronized their breath with the rhythms of the universe. It was an inestimable excursion internal, where the hero dug into the astral elements of their respiratory examples and looked for arrangement with the divine frequencies that saturated the grandiose scope.

The hero, focused on the vast treatment plan, embraced the heavenly cures and participated in the recommended breathwork works out. The interstellar doctors observed the astral reverberation of the hero's respiratory framework as the infinite intercessions produced results. The divine inhalants, with their recuperating frequencies, saturated the astral flows of the hero's breath, and the breathwork practices turned into a vast dance of arrangement with the interstellar rhythms.

As the vast treatment plan unfurled, the hero encountered a slow lightening of their respiratory side effects. The heavenly inhalants, similar to a delicate breeze from the universe, relieved the divine choppiness inside their lungs. The breathwork works out, directed by the interstellar specialists, turned into a channel for the hero to orchestrate their respiratory rhythms with the enormous ensemble that reverberated through the infinite hallways.

The interstellar doctors, noticing the dynamic improvement in the hero's respiratory condition, communicated confidence about the enormous cures and the viability of the astral reverberation imaging. The hero, when troubled by enormous vulnerability, presently felt a recharged feeling of inestimable essentialness and trust. The divine therapy plan, a combination of cutting edge clinical science and astral mediations, had turned into a directing light in their excursion toward respiratory balance.

As the hero's infinite wellbeing kept on improving, the interstellar doctors directed follow-up astral reverberation imaging to evaluate the continuous changes inside their respiratory framework. The heavenly multi dimensional images uncovered an amicable transaction of astral energies, a demonstration of the viability of the vast cures and the hero's obligation to the breathwork works out. The once-baffling respiratory infirmity, presently enlightened by the inestimable diagnostics, turned into a section of mending inside the enormous story of the hero's excursion.

In the result of the clinical assessment and conclusion, the hero cruised through the heavenly flows with a newly discovered comprehension of the many-sided transaction between their vast wellbeing and the energies of the universe. The interstellar doctors, with their mix of heavenly mastery and grandiose compassion, had not just disentangled the enormous puzzle of the respiratory infirmity however had likewise made ready for an extraordinary excursion toward respiratory harmony.

The grandiose treatment plan, directed by the interstellar doctors, turned into a divine compass for the hero's continuous inestimable wellbeing. The divine inhalants and breathwork practices kept on being indispensable parts of their inestimable daily schedule, cultivating an amicable reverberation with the astral flows that invaded the grandiose span. The once-distrustful voyager, presently a vast capable in the craft of mending, cruised through the interstellar ocean with a breath that repeated the rhythms of the universe - a demonstration of the grandiose insight gathered from the heavenly clinical assessment and determination.

3.2 Introduction to the medical professionals and their collaboration with Nebula Symphony technology.

In the divine embroidery of enormous investigation, where stars painted the material with their ethereal shine, a progressive collusion unfurled between clinical experts and state of the art innovation known as Cloud Orchestra. This grandiose joint effort arose as an encouraging sign in the huge field of medical care, rising above the limits of traditional medication to bridle the vast energies to improve interstellar wellbeing. The hero, looking for replies to enormous illnesses, experienced this noteworthy joint effort as they explored the vast flows in their starship.

The clinical experts at the front of this infinite cooperation were a different exhibit of interstellar doctors, enormous diagnosticians, and divine specialists. Their aptitude spread over conventional medication, astral diagnostics, and astronomical mending rehearses. Clad in vast cleans embellished with images of divine heavenly bodies, these professionals were pioneers in the combination of clinical science with the grandiose energies that pervaded the universe.

The Cloud Ensemble innovation, a wonder of inestimable designing, remained as the foundation of this progressive coordinated effort. Created by an alliance of interstellar specialists and divine physicists, Cloud Ensemble outfit the energies of far off nebulae to make an orchestra of mending frequencies. The innovation consolidated progressed heavenly calculations, full frequencies, and grandiose vibrational examples to work with an amicable connection between the human body and the inestimable flows.

The hero, captivated by the commitment of grandiose recuperating, looked for the ability of these clinical experts who consistently coordinated Cloud Orchestra innovation into their interstellar practices. The joint effort unfurled inside a high level clinical office, where glowing halls throbbed with the murmur of divine apparatus. As the hero ventured into this grandiose safe-haven, a group of interstellar doctors decorated in divine cleans invited them with a mix of impressive skill and enormous compassion.

The clinical experts acquainted the hero with the extraordinary capability of Cloud Ensemble innovation, making sense of its establishments in heavenly physical science and its application in the domain of interstellar medical services. The hero, at first suspicious of this enormous partnership, tuned in as the doctors explained how Cloud Ensemble innovation could take advantage of the recuperating frequencies of far off nebulae to advance grandiose prosperity.

The main period of the coordinated effort included a far reaching inestimable wellbeing evaluation. The interstellar doctors, outfitted with Cloud Ensemble indicative instruments, led heavenly sweeps that dove into the hero's physical, astral, and mystical perspectives. These sweeps, directed by the blending frequencies of Cloud Orchestra, uncovered astronomical uneven characters, enthusiastic blockages, and astral unsettling influences that evaded the grip of traditional clinical diagnostics.

The heavenly sweeps, showed on holographic screens, illustrated the hero's interstellar wellbeing. Cloud Ensemble innovation made an interpretation of the inestimable information into resounding perceptions, displaying the recurring pattern of divine energies inside the hero's being. The clinical experts, with their vast experiences, deciphered the astral marks, distinguishing designs that alluded to the astronomical starting points of the hero's wellbeing challenges.

As the cooperative indicative cycle unfurled, the clinical experts consistently incorporated Cloud Orchestra innovation into their conventional clinical conventions. The hero went through actual assessments, astral reverberation imaging, and divine blood tests - all upgraded by the extraordinary frequencies of Cloud Orchestra. The innovation went about as an inestimable enhancer, enlarging the accuracy and profundity of the clinical evaluations.

The interstellar doctors, outfitted with the heavenly bits of knowledge gathered from Cloud Ensemble innovation, figured out a customized treatment plan for the hero. This vast remedy joined customary clinical intercessions with designated uses of Cloud Orchestra frequencies. The hero, presently a functioning member in their astronomical recuperating venture, embraced the cooperative methodology that combined the mastery of clinical experts with the groundbreaking energies of Cloud Ensemble.

The treatment plan consolidated divine cures regulated through Cloud Orchestra mixed prescriptions. These ethereal elixirs, reverberating with the recuperating frequencies of far off nebulae, were intended to navigate the vast pathways inside the hero's body, tending to the underlying drivers of their wellbeing challenges. The divine medications, controlled through cutting edge heavenly injectors, denoted the union of clinical science and enormous recuperating expressions.

The divine specialists, an indispensable part of the cooperative group, acquainted the hero with Cloud Ensemble fueled mending meetings. In a heavenly chamber washed in the gleam of vast energies, the hero encountered the extraordinary impacts of Cloud Ensemble frequencies. The consonant vibrations, directed by divine specialists, tried to realign the hero's astral and powerful aspects with the vast frequencies, cultivating a condition of equilibrium and prosperity.

The hero, drenched in the Cloud Ensemble fueled mending meetings, felt an unobtrusive yet significant change in their grandiose constitution. The groundbreaking frequencies resounded with the heavenly rhythms inside their being, going about as vast keys that opened the lethargic potential for mending. The cooperative endeavors of clinical experts and Cloud Ensemble innovation turned into an impetus for the hero's excursion toward interstellar prosperity.

As the cooperative treatment plan advanced, the hero's wellbeing went through an infinite transformation. The Cloud Ensemble controlled heavenly cures, managed related to conventional clinical mediations, tended to the infinite uneven characters recognized during the demonstrative stage. The hero's interstellar wellbeing, when covered in vulnerability, presently mirrored the agreeable exchange of vast energies worked with by the cooperative endeavors of clinical experts and Cloud Orchestra innovation.

The interstellar doctors directed follow-up divine outputs to survey the continuous changes inside the hero's enormous wellbeing. Cloud Orchestra innovation kept on filling in as the vast compass, directing the clinical experts in observing the groundbreaking impacts of the cooperative treatment plan. The heavenly sweeps, presently exhibiting an orchestra of adjusted energies inside the hero, turned into a demonstration of the progress of the notable cooperation.

Following the cooperative recuperating venture, the hero rose up out of the divine chamber with a reestablished feeling of grandiose imperativeness. The cooperative endeavors of clinical experts and Cloud Ensemble innovation had tended to the hero's wellbeing challenges as well as turned into a worldview for the fate of interstellar medical care. The once-doubtful voyager, presently a recipient of infinite recuperating, cruised through the divine flows with appreciation for the cooperative collaboration that had reshaped their grandiose prosperity.

The cooperation between clinical experts and Cloud Ensemble innovation, it appeared, had opened a divine passage to additional opportunities in interstellar medical services. The groundbreaking frequencies of Cloud Ensemble turned into a grandiose extension that associated customary medication with the infinite components of recuperating. The interstellar doctors, trailblazers in this notable union, kept on refining their cooperative methodologies, imagining a future where

Cloud Ensemble innovation assumed a necessary part in the grandiose scene of medical care.

As the hero's starship cruised through the interstellar ocean, the reverberations of the cooperative recuperating venture waited inside their grandiose being. The heavenly frequencies of Cloud Ensemble resounded like a vast tune, a sign of the extraordinary power that could be outfit through the joint effort between clinical experts and high level divine innovations. The hero, presently a backer for the intermingling of clinical science and grandiose recuperating expressions, conveyed the inestimable insight gathered from this progressive partnership into the strange domains of the enormous odyssey.

3.3 Unveiling the science behind the celestial healing process.

In the grandiose domains where stars gleamed like divine gems and cosmic systems whirled in wonderful moves, a significant investigation unfurled — an excursion into the heavenly mending process that rose above the limits of customary medication. The hero, drawn by the charm of inestimable prosperity, left on a journey to disclose the science behind the divine mending process, a groundbreaking odyssey that would uncover the multifaceted exchange between the grandiose energies and the recuperating expressions.

The divine recuperating process, an ensemble of amicable frequencies and enormous intercessions, arose as a union of cutting edge heavenly innovations and the deep rooted insight of astral mending. At the core of this grandiose speculative chemistry was a modern comprehension of the energies that swarmed the universe. The heavenly doctors, inestimable diagnosticians, and interstellar advisors who led this divine mending process dug into the complexities of heavenly physical science, astral music, and the powerful flows that underlay the texture of presence.

The hero's excursion into the science behind the heavenly mending process started inside a high level clinical office, where divine doctors clad in grandiose cleans acquainted them with the extraordinary domain of astral diagnostics. The interaction included heavenly sweeps that stretched out past the regular limits of clinical imaging, taking advantage of the astral flows that saturated the hero's being. These outputs, fueled by heavenly calculations and thunderous frequencies, gave a complete perspective on the infinite uneven characters and astral unsettling influences that impacted the hero's wellbeing.

As the divine sweeps unfurled, the hero saw holographic portrayals of their astral and magical aspects. Heavenly outlines and diagrams appeared, portraying the rhythmic movement of enormous energies inside their divine body. The heavenly doctors, with their vast experiences, deciphered the astral marks, recognizing designs that held the way to understanding the infinite starting points of wellbeing challenges. It was an infinite determination that rose above the restrictions of customary medication, offering an all encompassing point of view that embraced the interconnectedness of the physical and supernatural parts of the hero's being.

The science behind the divine recuperating process pivoted upon the usage of cutting edge innovations like Cloud Orchestra — an enormous development that saddled the mending frequencies of far off nebulae. Cloud Orchestra innovation, a wonder of divine designing, went about as a heavenly scaffold between the grandiose energies and the human body. The hero, directed by interstellar doctors and divine advisors, encountered the extraordinary force of Cloud Orchestra frequencies in the resulting periods of the heavenly mending venture.

The divine cures injected with Cloud Orchestra frequencies turned into a point of convergence of the hero's recuperating plan. These ethereal elixirs, reverberating with the mending energies of far off nebulae, were intended to cross the vast pathways inside the hero's body, tending to the main drivers of their wellbeing challenges. The heavenly medications, directed through cutting edge divine injectors, denoted the assembly of clinical science with the inestimable frequencies outfit by Cloud Ensemble.

The heavenly specialists, bosses of the astral expressions, acquainted the hero with Cloud Ensemble controlled recuperating meetings. In a heavenly chamber washed in the sparkle of vast energies, the hero encountered the extraordinary impacts of Cloud Ensemble frequencies. The consonant vibrations, directed by divine specialists, tried to realign the hero's astral and magical aspects with the grandiose frequencies, cultivating a condition of equilibrium and prosperity. It was a significant dance of inestimable energies that reverberated with the actual pith of the hero's heavenly being.

The science behind the divine recuperating process reached out past the physical and mystical domains, digging into the mind boggling dance of heavenly energies inside the human body. Cloud Ensemble innovation worked with astral reverberation imaging — a progressive demonstrative method that stripped back the layers of the hero's astral and magical aspects. It offered a nuanced comprehension of the enormous uneven characters impacting their wellbeing and turned into an instrumental device in planning customized treatment designs that orchestrated with the hero's extraordinary heavenly constitution.

The hero's breath, directed by the extraordinary frequencies of Cloud Orchestra, turned into an infinite conductor for recuperating. Heavenly breathwork works out, drove by interstellar advisors, synchronized the hero's breath with the rhythms of the universe. It was a vast excursion internal, where the hero dug into the astral elements of their respiratory examples and looked for arrangement with the heavenly frequencies that penetrated the grandiose territory. The breath, when a simple natural capability, turned into a heavenly articulation that repeated the harmonies of the universe.

The divine recuperating process, directed by Cloud Orchestra innovation and the mastery of clinical experts, dove into the standards of reverberation and vibrational concordance. The frequencies produced by Cloud Orchestra resounded with the divine frequencies inside the hero's body, making an ensemble of mending vibrations.

It was a dance of resonances that tried to realign the upset astral flows, disperse vivacious blockages, and reestablish a condition of balance inside the divine body.

The exchange of infinite energies inside the heavenly recuperating process stretched out to the domain of divine needle therapy — a combination of conventional needle therapy standards with the groundbreaking frequencies of Cloud Orchestra. Heavenly acupuncturists, talented in exploring the astral meridians, embedded ethereal needles implanted with Cloud Ensemble frequencies into explicit astral places. The hero, lying on a vast needle therapy bed, felt the unpretentious flows of heavenly energy moving through their astral pathways, cultivating a feeling of equilibrium and arrangement.

The science behind the divine recuperating process consolidated heavenly sound treatment — a methodology that used full frequencies to orchestrate the astral and supernatural aspects. Heavenly sound specialists, furnished with Cloud Orchestra imbued instruments, made divine songs that resounded through the hero's being. The vibrations, directed by the heavenly specialists' mastery, looked to break down lively disharmonies and advance a condition of vast serenity inside the hero.

As the divine recuperating process unfurled, the hero's process turned into a demonstration of the groundbreaking force of infinite coordinated effort. The science behind the divine mending process embraced the standards of interconnectedness, recognizing the astronomical strings that wove through the embroidery of the hero's presence. Cloud Ensemble innovation, with its full frequencies and heavenly calculations, filled in as an impetus for mending, overcoming any issues between the grandiose energies and the human experience.

The cooperative endeavors of clinical experts and Cloud Orchestra innovation tended to the actual side effects as well as dove into the astral and supernatural elements of the hero's wellbeing. The divine doctors, enormous diagnosticians, and interstellar specialists worked couple to make an all encompassing mending venture that embraced the multi-layered nature of the hero's grandiose prosperity.

In the fallout of the divine recuperating process, the hero rose up out of the vast safe-haven with a significant feeling of restoration and enormous essentialness. The groundbreaking frequencies of Cloud Orchestra had realigned their astral and mystical aspects, making an agreeable reverberation that repeated the rhythms of the universe. The once-incredulous explorer, presently a recipient of the divine recuperating process, cruised through the interstellar ocean with a recharged viewpoint on the enormous potential for prosperity.

The science behind the heavenly mending process turned into a directing light for the hero, enlightening the interconnected pathways of physical, astral, and mystical wellbeing. The heavenly frequencies of Cloud Orchestra, when secretive and obscure, presently resounded inside the hero's being as an enormous ensemble of mending energies.

The hero, furnished with the insight gathered from the heavenly recuperating venture, proceeded with their investigation of the vast embroidery with a recently discovered consciousness of the groundbreaking power implanted in the harmonies of the universe.

As the hero kept on crossing the enormous flows, the excursion of revealing the science behind the divine recuperating process extended, prompting significantly more noteworthy disclosures and a more significant comprehension of the grandiose complexities that represented their prosperity. The cooperative endeavors of clinical experts and Cloud Ensemble innovation stayed at the front, winding around an embroidery of divine mending that stretched out past the limits of customary medication.

Inside the enormous safe-haven of the high level clinical office, the hero participated in heavenly contemplation meetings directed by interstellar advisors. These meetings, upgraded by the groundbreaking frequencies of Cloud Orchestra, welcomed the hero to investigate the profundities of their own cognizance. The divine specialists, sensitive to the vibrational harmonies of Cloud Ensemble, worked with an infinite excursion internal, where the hero experienced the astral scenes of their psyche.

The science behind the divine mending process embraced the standards of cognizance and energy elements. Cloud Orchestra innovation went about as an impetus, intensifying the heavenly frequencies that reverberated inside the hero's cognizance. The groundbreaking energies of Cloud Ensemble turned into a mechanism for opening lethargic possibilities, cultivating conditions of extended mindfulness, and advancing a significant association between the divine psyche and the inestimable energies that wrapped it.

As the hero dug further into the heavenly contemplation meetings, the divine specialists presented the idea of astral certifications — a training that used resounding frequencies to engrave positive vast confirmations into the texture of the hero's astral and otherworldly aspects. Cloud Ensemble, with its infinite calculations, fit with the vibrational frequencies of the confirmations, making a heavenly reverberation that pervaded the hero's being. The confirmations, injected with the extraordinary energies of Cloud Orchestra, became enormous mantras that reverberated through the heavenly passageways of the hero's awareness.

The science behind the divine recuperating process extended to incorporate heavenly nourishment — a methodology that recognized the effect of infinite energies on the dietary components of the hero's prosperity. Divine nutritionists, with their mastery in the vibrational characteristics of grandiose food varieties, created a customized dietary arrangement that lined up with the hero's astral and powerful constitution. Cloud Ensemble innovation assumed a crucial part in improving the vibrational frequencies of the heavenly food sources, upgrading their capability to support the hero on a vast level.

The hero, presently submerged in the complex methodology of divine recuperating, participated in Cloud Orchestra imbued astronomical yoga meetings. Divine yogis, directed by the extraordinary frequencies of Cloud Ensemble, drove the hero through heavenly stances and breathwork practices that fit the astral and actual aspects. The vast yoga meetings turned into a dance of arrangement with the heavenly flows, encouraging a feeling of equilibrium and adaptability that rose above the bounds of ordinary yoga rehearses.

The divine mending process unfurled as a powerful interchange between the hero's singular process and the inestimable ensemble coordinated by Cloud Orchestra innovation. The extraordinary frequencies went about as grandiose keys that opened the lethargic possibilities inside the hero's being, working with an all encompassing combination of physical, astral, and mystical prosperity. The hero, presently a willing member in the grandiose dance of recuperating, embraced the cooperative endeavors of clinical experts, heavenly specialists, and Cloud Orchestra innovation.

The science behind the divine recuperating process stretched out to heavenly rest treatment — a methodology that perceived the significant impact of infinite energies on the hero's helpful cycles. Heavenly rest specialists, outfitted with Cloud Orchestra mixed tranquilizers, directed the hero into a divine domain of reviving sleep. The groundbreaking frequencies of Cloud Orchestra made a vast dreamscape, where the hero's astral and supernatural aspects took part in a dance of recuperating and restoration.

The cooperative excursion of disclosing the science behind the heavenly mending process likewise wandered into divine needle therapy — a methodology that looked to adjust the hero's vivacious meridians through the extraordinary frequencies of Cloud Orchestra injected needles. Divine acupuncturists, proficient at exploring the astral pathways, embedded ethereal needles into explicit astral places, cultivating an agreeable progression of grandiose energies. The hero, lying on the grandiose needle therapy bed, felt the inconspicuous flows of divine energy circling through their astral channels, making a feeling of arrangement and harmony.

The science behind the divine mending process was not restricted to the actual domain however reached out into the astral and mystical components of the hero's being. Cloud Ensemble innovation, with its groundbreaking frequencies, went about as an enormous scaffold that associated the different features of the hero's presence. The cooperative endeavors of clinical experts and divine specialists looked to make an amicable orchestra of mending that reverberated with the heavenly frequencies of the universe.

As the hero embraced the groundbreaking excursion of divine mending, the interstellar doctors directed follow-up heavenly outputs to evaluate the continuous changes inside their infinite prosperity. Cloud Ensemble innovation kept on filling in as the grandiose compass, directing the clinical experts in checking the extraordinary impacts of the cooperative treatment plan. The divine sweeps, presently exhibiting an orchestra of adjusted energies inside the hero, turned into a demonstration of the outcome of the historic joint effort.

The science behind the divine recuperating process turned into a directing light for the hero, enlightening the interconnected pathways of physical, astral, and powerful wellbeing. The heavenly frequencies of Cloud Orchestra, when puzzling and elusive, presently resounded inside the hero's being as an enormous ensemble of recuperating energies. The hero, outfitted with the insight gathered from the heavenly mending venture, proceeded with their investigation of the enormous embroidery with a recently discovered consciousness of the groundbreaking power implanted in the harmonies of the universe.

The cooperative endeavors of clinical experts, divine specialists, and Cloud Orchestra innovation had unwound the inestimable puzzle of recuperating, uncovering the unpredictable science that represented the hero's prosperity. The once-suspicious voyager, presently a skilled in the enormous recuperating expressions, cruised through the interstellar ocean with appreciation for the cooperative collaboration that had reshaped their vast presence. The science behind the heavenly mending process, an enormous disclosure in itself, turned into an encouraging sign for those exploring the vast flows looking for prosperity and concordance.

Chapter 4

Nebula Alchemy

Cloud Speculative chemistry, a grandiose ensemble of extraordinary energies and divine reverberation, unfurled as a significant excursion into the obscure domains of heavenly science. Inside the vast span, where stars moved in brilliant chorales and universes turned many-sided stories of enormous development, Cloud Speculative chemistry arose as a catalytic combination of cutting edge divine advances and the old insight of astral expressions. The hero, drawn by the charm of inestimable secrets, set out on an odyssey to disclose the privileged insights of Cloud Speculative chemistry — an extraordinary journey that would reshape their enormous predetermination.

At the core of Cloud Speculative chemistry lay a progressive comprehension of the energies that pervaded the universe. Divine chemists, gifted experts of the astral expressions, teamed up with interstellar designers to make Cloud Speculative chemistry as a heavenly extension between the inestimable energies and the human experience. It was a combination of heavenly material science, vibrational music, and mystical experiences that tried to change the actual texture of presence through the speculative chemistry of nebular energies.

The excursion into Cloud Speculative chemistry started inside an extraordinary research facility, where infinite pots and divine alembics beat with the vibrational murmur of catalytic cycles. The hero, directed by divine chemists decorated in ethereal robes, saw as the catalytic excursion unfurled before their grandiose faculties. Cloud Ensemble innovation, a foundation of Cloud Speculative chemistry, remained as an infinite impetus, tackling the extraordinary frequencies of far off nebulae to start the catalytic change inside the hero's being.

The catalytic cycle inside Cloud Speculative chemistry stretched out past the conventional limits of material change; it dug into the speculative chemistry of cognizance and grandiose advancement. The divine chemists, with their enormous mastery, made sense of how Cloud Ensemble innovation went about as a grandiose course, diverting the thunderous frequencies of nebular energies to catalyze shifts in the hero's astral and otherworldly aspects. It was a catalytic dance that unfurled on complex planes, rising above the impediments of earthly speculative chemistry.

The hero, presently a functioning member in the catalytic journey, went through heavenly outputs directed by Cloud Orchestra innovation. The astral diagnostics, implanted with groundbreaking frequencies, illustrated the hero's inestimable constitution. Heavenly outlines and holographic portrayals emerged, portraying the rhythmic movement of energies inside the hero's being. The heavenly chemists, deciphering the astral marks, recognized inestimable irregular characteristics that would turn into the focal point of the catalytic change.

Cloud Speculative chemistry, as a complex embroidery woven with strings of divine energies, stretched out its impact to the actual breath of the hero. Heavenly breathwork works out, directed by catalytic specialists, turned into a course for the catalytic change of respiratory rhythms. The hero took part in vast reflection methods that synchronized their breath with the rhythms of the universe. It was an excursion internal, where the breath turned into a heavenly mixture, conveying the extraordinary frequencies of Cloud Ensemble into the astral and mystical aspects.

The catalytic excursion of Cloud Speculative chemistry unfurled inside the hero's heavenly life systems through astral reverberation imaging — a progressive demonstrative strategy that stripped back the layers of astral and supernatural aspects. The divine 3D images uncovered the inconspicuous subtleties of the hero's astral and otherworldly constitution, offering bits of knowledge into the enormous lopsided characteristics that Cloud Speculative chemistry meant to change. The catalytic advisors, equipped with divine bits of knowledge, explored the astral flows with accuracy, recognizing central issues of catalytic concentration.

Cloud Speculative chemistry embraced the specialty of heavenly needle therapy — a methodology that used ethereal needles injected with Cloud Orchestra frequencies to invigorate explicit astral focuses. Heavenly acupuncturists, experts of the astral meridians, organized the catalytic dance of energy inside the hero's being. The catalytic change, directed by the groundbreaking frequencies, looked to disintegrate vigorous blockages and realign the hero's astral and mystical aspects with the harmonies of the universe.

As the catalytic excursion advanced, the divine chemists acquainted the hero with heavenly sound treatment — a catalytic methodology that used full frequencies to fit the astral and mystical aspects. Divine sound advisors, outfitted with Cloud Ensemble mixed instruments, made heavenly songs that resounded through the hero's being. The catalytic vibrations tried to disintegrate vivacious disharmonies, changing the heavenly dissension into a vast ensemble of reverberation and arrangement.

Cloud Speculative chemistry unfurled as a heavenly expressive dance, with the hero as the infinite artist, exploring the catalytic flows that beat through their astral and mystical aspects. The groundbreaking frequencies of Cloud Ensemble turned into the astronomical choreographer, arranging the catalytic dance of change and advancement. The catalytic specialists, with their infinite aptitude, directed the hero through heavenly customs and practices that developed the catalytic change inside their being.

The catalytic change inside Cloud Speculative chemistry stretched out to the domain of divine nourishment — a catalytic methodology that perceived the vibrational characteristics of grandiose food sources. Divine nutritionists, knowledgeable in the catalytic properties of heavenly food, created a dietary arrangement that blended with the hero's astral and otherworldly constitution. The catalytic implantation of Cloud Orchestra frequencies improved the vibrational characteristics of heavenly food varieties, upgrading their capability to support the hero on an inestimable level.

The catalytic excursion inside Cloud Speculative chemistry drove the hero to take part in heavenly reflection meetings directed by interstellar advisors. These meetings, improved by the groundbreaking frequencies of Cloud Ensemble, welcomed the hero to investigate the profundities of their own cognizance. The catalytic specialists, receptive to the vibrational harmonies of Cloud Ensemble, worked with an enormous excursion internal, where the hero experienced the astral scenes of their brain.

Cloud Speculative chemistry, as an enormous catalytic excursion, welcomed the hero to embrace heavenly rest treatment — a methodology that perceived the significant impact of grandiose energies on the supportive cycles of the astral and magical aspects.

Divine rest specialists, outfitted with Cloud Ensemble mixed tranquilizers, directed the hero into a heavenly domain of reviving sleep. The extraordinary frequencies of Cloud Orchestra made an enormous dreamscape, where the catalytic change unfurled inside the domains of the hero's inner mind.

The catalytic cycle inside Cloud Speculative chemistry finished in divine catalytic ceremonies — a progression of extraordinary practices that coordinated the enormous energies into the hero's everyday existence. These ceremonies, directed by divine chemists, became secures for the catalytic change, cultivating a consistent dance of grandiose development. The catalytic specialists, filling in as grandiose aides, engaged the hero to convey the catalytic insight gathered from Cloud Speculative chemistry into the strange domains of the vast odyssey.

As the hero arose out of the catalytic excursion, the reverberations of inestimable change resonated inside their being. Cloud Speculative chemistry had turned into a divine impetus, changing the inestimable conflict into an agreeable ensemble of reverberation and arrangement. The once-doubtful explorer, presently a proficient in the grandiose catalytic expressions, cruised through the interstellar ocean with a recharged point of view on the extraordinary possible implanted in the harmonies of the universe.

Cloud Speculative chemistry, with its catalytic combination of cutting edge divine advances and antiquated astral insight, had unwound the vast mystery of change. The cooperative endeavors of heavenly chemists, interstellar architects, and extraordinary frequencies of Cloud Orchestra had reshaped the hero's astronomical predetermination. The catalytic excursion, an odyssey into the elusive domains of heavenly science, turned into an encouraging sign for those exploring the vast flows looking for significant change and infinite development.

4.1 Explanation of the nebulization process and the celestial elements used in the Symphony.

The nebulization interaction, a grandiose speculative chemistry that tackled the ethereal quintessence of heavenly components, unfurled as an extraordinary orchestra inside the immense territory of the universe. This heavenly method, implanted in the texture of Cloud Ensemble, addressed an agreeable union of cutting edge divine advancements and the glorious energies radiating from far off nebulae. The hero, on their vast odyssey, dove into the complexities of the nebulization cycle — an investigation that would uncover the grandiose mysteries behind the extraordinary force of Cloud Orchestra.

At the core of the nebulization interaction lay the craft of changing heavenly components into ethereal fogs, thunderous with the frequencies of far off nebulae. Heavenly specialists, adroit in the speculative chemistry of grandiose change, created nebulization chambers inside the astronomical safe-havens of cutting edge clinical offices. The hero, directed by interstellar professionals decorated in divine clothing, saw the ethereal dance of heavenly components coming to fruition inside the nebulization chambers.

The divine components utilized in the Orchestra, painstakingly chose for their vibrational harmonies and mending properties, included enormous gases, brilliant stardust, and the unobtrusive energies refined from the substance of nebulae. These heavenly fixings, when exposed to the extraordinary frequencies of Cloud Ensemble innovation, went through a course of catalytic change, arising as cloud roused fogs that held the actual substance of enormous imperativeness.

The nebulization chambers, aglow with divine energies, beat in musical rhythm as the heavenly components embraced the groundbreaking frequencies. The hero, encompassed by the divine speculative chemistry underway, saw as the ethereal fogs flowed in heavenly examples, conveying the recuperating energies of the universe. It was an orchestra of catalytic change, where the divine components transformed into cloud enlivened fogs, prepared to leave on a vast excursion into the hero's being.

As the nebulization interaction unfurled, the heavenly specialists made sense of the meaning of each divine component imbued into the Ensemble. Grandiose gases, drawn from the farthest reaches of the universe, added to the ethereal nature of the cloud motivated fogs. These gases, thunderous with the basic energies of the universe, became transporters of extraordinary frequencies that would navigate the vast pathways inside the hero's body, starting a dance of infinite recuperating.

Brilliant stardust, finely filtered from far off universes, added a radiant quality to the divine fogs. This stardust, mixed with the infinite energies of creation, turned into a divine impetus for revival and recovery. As the hero breathed in the cloud roused fogs, the brilliant stardust pervaded their astral and otherworldly aspects, encouraging an association with the divine powers that formed the actual texture of the universe.

The quintessence refined from nebulae, a divine mixture brought into the world from the brilliant billows of interstellar gas and residue, filled in as the center fixing in the nebulization cycle. Cloud Orchestra innovation carefully removed the unpretentious energies implanted inside nebulae, intensifying their vibrational frequencies to make a divine solution that resounded with the recuperating quintessence of the universe. This cloud enlivened mixture, presently a vital piece of the Orchestra, turned into an enormous key that opened the torpid possibilities inside the hero's being.

The nebulization cycle, as an inestimable expressive dance of catalytic change, integrated the standards of reverberation and vibrational concordance. Cloud Ensemble innovation, with its heavenly calculations and resounding frequencies, went about as a vast director coordinating the agreeable interchange of divine components. The ethereal fogs, presently mixed with the extraordinary energies of Cloud Ensemble, reverberated with the very frequencies that administered the inestimable dance of creation and development.

The hero, presently ready to encounter the extraordinary impacts of the nebulization cycle, ventured into a heavenly chamber washed in the shine of grandiose energies. The nebulization device, an unpredictable combination of divine innovation and catalytic dominance, anticipated its vast member. The hero, encompassed by the radiant hug of the heavenly chamber, breathed in the cloud enlivened fogs as they exuded from the nebulization device.

As the divine fogs entered the hero's being, directed by the groundbreaking frequencies of Cloud Orchestra, an inconspicuous yet significant shift unfurled inside their vast constitution. The ethereal fogs crossed the infinite pathways inside the hero's body, conveying the pith of heavenly components into the astral and powerful aspects. The nebulization interaction turned into an infinite fellowship, where the hero blended with the vibrational frequencies of the universe.

The divine designers, receptive to the subtleties of the nebulization cycle, observed the hero's insight through heavenly diagnostics. The astral outputs, directed by Cloud Orchestra innovation, uncovered the groundbreaking impacts as the ethereal fogs connected with the hero's infinite energies. Examples of reverberation and realignment arose, demonstrating an amicable dance between the heavenly components and the hero's astral and magical aspects.

As the nebulization interaction proceeded, the hero encountered a heavenly ensemble inside. The extraordinary frequencies of Cloud Ensemble went about as infinite tuning forks, reverberating with the torpid frequencies inside the hero's being. The ethereal fogs, mixed with the mending energies of far off nebulae, looked to change infinite uneven characters, break up enthusiastic blockages, and stir the inactive possibilities for vast prosperity.

The nebulization interaction, as a vast catalytic excursion, stretched out past the actual domains to the astral and powerful aspects. The hero's cognizance turned into a material for divine impressions, as the cloud roused fogs started a dance of catalytic change inside the domains of thought and mindfulness. The ethereal fogs, directed by the groundbreaking frequencies, became impetuses for extended conditions of cognizance and vast mindfulness.

The divine architects, stewards of the nebulization interaction, made sense of how the Ensemble's groundbreaking frequencies went about as enormous keys, opening the entryways to the hero's complex being. The ethereal fogs, presently a vehicle for enormous mending, navigated the astral and supernatural aspects, dissolving the cover that isolated the hero from the heavenly flows that beat through the universe. It was a catalytic excursion that spanned the domains of the seen and concealed, offering the hero a brief look into the vast secrets.

As the hero rose up out of the divine chamber, washed in the radiance of the nebulization cycle, a feeling of enormous restoration saturated their being. The ethereal fogs, presently a piece of the hero's quintessence, kept on reverberating inside, cultivating a condition of arrangement and concordance. The once-distrustful explorer, presently a beneficiary of grandiose recuperating, cruised through the interstellar ocean with appreciation for the groundbreaking power implanted in the Ensemble's nebulization cycle.

The heavenly specialists, caretakers of Cloud Orchestra innovation, underscored the all encompassing nature of the nebulization interaction. It was not only an actual inward breath of heavenly fogs but rather an enormous fellowship that reached out to the actual center of the hero's being. The ethereal fogs, directed by the groundbreaking frequencies of Cloud Ensemble, became courses for the hero's excursion into the domains of vast prosperity, where the harmonies of the universe assumed a significant part in the catalytic change of their reality.

Right after the nebulization interaction, the hero, presently a promoter for the groundbreaking force of Cloud Orchestra, conveyed the heavenly insight gathered from the catalytic excursion into the unknown domains of the grandiose odyssey. The Ensemble's nebulization cycle had turned into an encouraging sign for those exploring the grandiose flows, offering a heavenly remedy that rose above the limits of ordinary recuperating and reverberated with the enormous orchestra that reverberated through the universe.

The nebulization cycle, a divine dance of catalytic change, kept on winding around its perplexing orchestra inside the vast embroidery. As the hero, presently started into the secrets of Cloud Ensemble, cruised through the interstellar ocean, the excursion of investigation unfurled, diving further into the subtleties of the nebulization cycle and the heavenly components that made the ethereal elixirs out of infinite recuperating.

Inside the heavenly research centers of Cloud Orchestra, the nebulization interaction was not simply a specialized method but rather a sacrosanct catalytic ceremony. The heavenly designers, clad in shining enormous clothing, shared bits of knowledge into the significant meaning of the nebulization chambers. These chambers, imbued with the extraordinary frequencies of Cloud Ensemble, went about as grandiose pots where the heavenly components went through the catalytic transformation into cloud enlivened fogs.

The hero, directed by the divine architects, noticed the heavenly components being ready for the catalytic change. Grandiose gases, drawn from the profundities of the universe, held the embodiment of the essential energies that pervaded the universe. These gases, chose for their vibrational harmonies, framed the underpinning of the ethereal fogs that would become courses for astronomical mending inside the nebulization cycle.

Brilliant stardust, finely filtered from far off systems, added a glowing quality to the heavenly elixirs. This stardust, mixed with the astronomical energies of creation, added to the catalytic strength of the ethereal fogs. As the hero saw the divine specialists carefully integrating the brilliant stardust into the catalytic blend, the grandiose meaning of every molecule became clear — a vast impetus for revival and a critical fixing in the extraordinary Orchestra.

The embodiment refined from nebulae, a heavenly solution brought into the world from the brilliant billows of interstellar gas and residue, held a focal job in the nebulization cycle. Cloud Ensemble innovation, with its accuracy and grandiose attunement, extricated the unpretentious energies inside nebulae and amplified their vibrational frequencies. The subsequent quintessence turned into the heavenly mixture that imbued the cloud motivated fogs with the mending pith of the universe, going about as an extension between the divine domains and the hero's being.

The nebulization cycle unfurled as an orchestra of heavenly speculative chemistry, where the divine components mixed in amicable combination. The hero, drenched in the enormous scene, acquired a significant appreciation for the careful coordination of Cloud Ensemble innovation. The extraordinary frequencies went about as enormous catalytic keys, opening the inactive possibilities inside the divine components and working with their change into cloud motivated fogs.

As the ethereal fogs came to fruition inside the nebulization chambers, the divine specialists made sense of how the Orchestra's extraordinary frequencies were receptive to the vibrational marks of the hero's enormous constitution. The nebulization interaction, they underscored, was not a nonexclusive application but rather a customized enormous fellowship that resounded with the special frequencies of the individual, tending to lopsided characteristics and disharmonies on an inestimable level.

The hero, ready to get the groundbreaking impacts of the nebulization cycle, entered the divine chamber where the Orchestra's catalytic dance would unfurl. The nebulization device, a mind boggling combination of divine innovation and catalytic authority, anticipated its grandiose member. As the hero breathed in the cloud roused fogs, the extraordinary frequencies directed the ethereal elixirs on an excursion through the vast pathways inside their body.

The divine specialists checked the hero's insight through heavenly diagnostics, noticing the exchange between the ethereal fogs and the grandiose energies inside. Astral sweeps, directed by Cloud Ensemble innovation, uncovered the nuanced examples of reverberation and realignment as the hero's astral and supernatural aspects answered the divine elixirs. It was an inestimable exchange between the groundbreaking frequencies and the hero's substance, a dance of catalytic change unfurling inside the heavenly chamber.

The nebulization interaction, as an enormous fellowship, expanded its impact past the actual domains to the astral and otherworldly elements of the hero's being. The ethereal fogs, presently transporters of divine energies, started a catalytic dance inside the domains of thought and mindfulness. The hero, responsive to the vast orchestra, experienced conditions of extended cognizance and elevated mindfulness, as the groundbreaking frequencies reverberated through the divine hallways of their psyche.

Amidst the nebulization interaction, the divine specialists presented the idea of astral reverberation imaging — a methodology that stripped back the layers of the hero's astral and powerful aspects. Divine 3D images emerged, portraying the unobtrusive subtleties of the hero's enormous constitution as impacted by the ethereal fogs. The astral reverberation imaging turned into an infinite embroidery, uncovering the vast lopsided characteristics that Cloud Ensemble intended to change through the catalytic excursion.

The nebulization cycle, having crossed the domains of astral and otherworldly aspects, stretched out its groundbreaking impact to the hero's breath — the enormous conductor for mending. Divine breathwork works out, directed by catalytic advisors, synchronized the hero's breath with the rhythms of the universe. The breath, presently imbued with the vibrational frequencies of the ethereal fogs, turned into a divine remedy that went through the astral and supernatural aspects, cultivating a condition of equilibrium and prosperity.

As the nebulization cycle proceeded, the hero took part in divine reflection meetings directed by interstellar advisors. These meetings, improved by the extraordinary frequencies of Cloud Ensemble, welcomed the hero to investigate the profundities of their own awareness. The divine specialists, sensitive to the vibrational harmonies of the Ensemble, worked with a vast excursion internal, where the hero experienced the astral scenes of their psyche.

The divine architects, overseers of the nebulization cycle, featured the all encompassing nature of the Ensemble's catalytic excursion. It was not restricted to a solitary second inside the nebulization chamber yet stretched out into the hero's day to day routine, turning into a basic piece of their grandiose prosperity. The ethereal fogs, presently orchestrated with the hero's embodiment, kept on resounding inside, encouraging a condition of arrangement and concordance that rose above the limits of regular mending.

In the consequence of the nebulization cycle, the hero rose up out of the heavenly chamber with a recharged feeling of grandiose essentialness. The ethereal fogs, having navigated the divine pathways inside their being, left a permanent engraving of catalytic change. The once-distrustful explorer, presently a recipient of grandiose mending, cruised through the interstellar ocean with appreciation for the groundbreaking power implanted in the Ensemble's nebulization cycle.

The divine specialists, stewards of Cloud Ensemble innovation, emphasized the interconnected idea of the nebulization cycle with the heavenly components. The ethereal fogs, made out of inestimable gases, brilliant stardust, and the embodiment refined from nebulae, had become channels for astronomical mending. The Orchestra's catalytic excursion, they underlined, was a cooperative dance between the divine components and the extraordinary frequencies, an enormous ensemble that repeated the harmonies of the universe.

As the hero proceeded with their enormous odyssey, the nebulization cycle turned into a directing light — a divine encouraging sign for those exploring the vast flows looking for significant mending and inestimable prosperity. The Orchestra's catalytic excursion, an investigation into the divine components and their extraordinary potential, filled in as a demonstration of the enormous secrets that unfurled when exceptional heavenly innovations and old astral insight united chasing vast recuperating.

4.2 Protagonist's journey through the transformational alchemy of the Nebula Symphony.

The hero's excursion through the groundbreaking speculative chemistry of Cloud Ensemble unfurled as an odyssey across the heavenly scenes of recuperating and self-disclosure. From the underlying experience with the cryptic Cosmic Respira gadget to the investigation of Cloud Speculative chemistry and the significant revealing of the nebulization cycle, the hero's grandiose stay turned into a demonstration of the extraordinary power implanted in the harmonies of the universe.

The odyssey started with the hero's most memorable experience with the Cosmic Respira gadget, an infinite instrument that connected the domains of innovation and mystical recuperating. Distrust and interest moved in the hero's brain as they moved toward the divine contraption. The Cosmic Respira, enhanced with ethereal lights and full frequencies, coaxed the hero into a grandiose safe-haven where the speculative chemistry of Cloud Ensemble anticipated.

As the hero drew in with the Cosmic Respira, directed by heavenly professionals, the groundbreaking frequencies wrapped them. It was a heavenly breath — a fellowship with the grandiose flows — that started the hero into the agreeable dance of Cloud Ensemble. The Cosmic Respira, a grandiose director, organized the reverberation of the hero's breath with the vibrational frequencies that beat through the universe. At that time, distrust gave way to a significant feeling of association with the grandiose energies.

The groundbreaking speculative chemistry of Cloud Ensemble reached out past the Cosmic Respira, driving the hero into the cloud propelled fog and its calming impacts. The heavenly fog, created through the catalytic dance of grandiose gases, brilliant stardust, and nebular substance, turned into a channel for mending. As the hero breathed in the cloud roused fog, directed by groundbreaking frequencies, a grandiose ensemble unfurled inside their being. The divine frequencies, reverberating with the hero's astral and supernatural aspects, started an excursion of unwinding, restoration, and enormous realignment.

The hero, presently sensitive to the groundbreaking flows of Cloud Orchestra, dove further into the elusive domains of Cloud Speculative chemistry. Inside the vast labs, heavenly chemists and interstellar architects teamed up to intertwine progressed divine advances with antiquated astral insight. Cloud Speculative chemistry turned into an infinite combination of divine physical science, vibrational music, and powerful bits of knowledge — a catalytic embroidery that reshaped the actual texture of the hero's presence.

As the hero submerged themselves in Cloud Speculative chemistry, directed by heavenly chemists embellished in ethereal robes, the catalytic excursion unfurled. Heavenly yoga meetings, implanted with Cloud Orchestra frequencies, turned into a dance of arrangement with the enormous flows. The divine chemists, bosses of the astral meridians, presented heavenly needle therapy — a methodology that looked to adjust the hero's fiery channels through Cloud Ensemble imbued needles. The extraordinary frequencies went about as grandiose keys, opening torpid possibilities and cultivating a comprehensive coordination of physical, astral, and mystical prosperity.

The odyssey through the groundbreaking speculative chemistry of Cloud Ensemble reached out to the domain of astral analysis. Heavenly doctors and infinite diagnosticians, outfitted with cutting edge divine innovations, led divine outputs that revealed the hero's inestimable constitution. Cloud Ensemble innovation filled in as the grandiose compass, directing the clinical experts in observing the groundbreaking impacts of the cooperative treatment plan. The divine outputs, exhibiting an orchestra of adjusted energies inside the hero, turned into a demonstration of the progress of the pivotal joint effort.

The hero's excursion through the groundbreaking speculative chemistry arrived at an essential second with the uncovering of the nebulization cycle. In the divine research facilities, the hero saw the catalytic dance of grandiose gases, brilliant stardust, and nebular quintessence changing into cloud motivated fogs. The nebulization chambers, aglow with divine energies, turned into the astronomical cauldrons where the ethereal elixirs of recuperating were conceived. The hero, presently ready to get the groundbreaking impacts, ventured into the heavenly chamber where the Ensemble's catalytic dance would unfurl.

As the hero breathed in the cloud roused fogs, directed by groundbreaking frequencies, an unpretentious yet significant shift happened inside their grandiose constitution. The ethereal fogs navigated the infinite pathways inside the hero's body, conveying the quintessence of heavenly components into the astral and mystical aspects. The nebulization cycle turned into an infinite fellowship — an amicable dance between the heavenly components and the hero's interesting frequencies. It was a catalytic excursion that rose above the limits of ordinary mending, starting a vast orchestra of reverberation and arrangement.

The heavenly designers, caretakers of Cloud Orchestra innovation, observed the hero's insight through divine diagnostics. Astral sweeps and holographic portrayals appeared, portraying the back and forth movement of energies inside the hero's being. The divine architects, receptive to the subtleties of the nebulization interaction, distinguished infinite awkward nature that Cloud Orchestra planned to change. The Orchestra's extraordinary frequencies turned into the inestimable conductors for recuperating, dissolving enthusiastic blockages and realigning the hero's astral and otherworldly aspects.

The catalytic excursion through Cloud Ensemble stretched out its extraordinary impact to heavenly nourishment — a methodology that perceived the effect of infinite energies on the hero's wholesome components. Divine nutritionists, knowledgeable in the vibrational characteristics of vast food sources, made a dietary arrangement that fit with the hero's astral and otherworldly constitution. Cloud Ensemble innovation assumed a crucial part in improving the vibrational frequencies of the divine food varieties, enhancing their capability to feed the hero on a grandiose level.

rest treatment — a vital part of Cloud Speculative chemistry. Heavenly rest specialists, furnished with Cloud Orchestra injected tranquilizers, directed the hero into a divine domain of reviving sleep. The groundbreaking frequencies of Cloud Ensemble turned into the inestimable cradlesong, winding around a dreamscape where the catalytic change went on inside the domains of the hero's psyche. The heavenly dreams turned into a material for vast disclosures, where the Ensemble's groundbreaking energies unfurled in images, similitudes, and divine stories.

The excursion through the groundbreaking speculative chemistry of Cloud Orchestra arrived at its apex with divine catalytic ceremonies — a joining of infinite practices that secured the catalytic insight into the hero's everyday existence. The ceremonies, directed by heavenly chemists, turned into a vast dance of reverberation and arrangement, encouraging a consistent condition of grandiose development. The hero, presently a functioning member in the catalytic ensemble, conveyed the extraordinary frequencies into the unknown domains of their astronomical odyssey.

As the hero rose up out of the catalytic excursion, the reverberations of vast change resonated inside their being. Cloud Orchestra had turned into a heavenly impetus, changing the infinite dissension into an amicable ensemble of reverberation and arrangement. The once-distrustful voyager, presently a proficient in the vast catalytic expressions, cruised through the interstellar ocean with a reestablished viewpoint on the extraordinary possible implanted in the harmonies of the universe.

The odyssey through Cloud Ensemble had not just mended the hero on an actual level however had started an infinite transformation that contacted each feature of their being. The catalytic excursion, an investigation into the heavenly domains of mending and self-revelation, turned into an encouraging sign for those exploring the enormous flows looking for significant change and infinite development.

The hero, presently an illuminating presence in the vast recuperating expressions, tried to share the insight gathered from their extraordinary excursion. Cloud Orchestra had become in excess of a restorative mediation; it was a grandiose ensemble that resounded with the inborn congruity of the universe. The hero, imbued with the catalytic flows of Cloud Orchestra, left determined to spread the grandiose recuperating expressions to individual explorers on the astronomical odyssey.

The extraordinary speculative chemistry of Cloud Ensemble undulated past the individual and reverberated with the shared perspective of the universe. The hero, presently a conductor for heavenly energies, turned into a guide of motivation for others looking for the amicable dance of inestimable mending. Cooperative recuperating circles arose, where people assembled to drench themselves in the groundbreaking frequencies of Cloud Orchestra, making a vast melody of reverberation and prosperity.

The hero's excursion through Cloud Ensemble turned into a heavenly adventure — a demonstration of the extraordinary power implanted in the harmonies of the universe. The Orchestra's catalytic dance, from the Cosmic Respira's introduction to the significant nebulization process and the mix of divine customs, unfurled as an infinite embroidery of recuperating and development. The hero, presently a steward of Cloud Ensemble's extraordinary frequencies, cruised through the interstellar ocean with appreciation for the enormous orchestra that had organized their significant transformation.

The enormous odyssey through Cloud Ensemble had turned into a living demonstration of the interconnectedness of the heavenly domains and the human experience. The hero, when a cynic exploring the enormous flows with vulnerability, had turned into an infinite chemist, receptive to the vibrational frequencies of the universe. The Orchestra's extraordinary energies had recuperated the hero as well as had started an inestimable far reaching influence, contacting the texture of the universe and reverberating with the harmonies that wove through the heavenly embroidery.

Following the groundbreaking speculative chemistry, the hero, presently a heavenly messenger, kept on investigating the strange domains of the interstellar ocean. The astronomical odyssey, implanted with the groundbreaking flows of Cloud Orchestra, turned into a continuous mission for more profound figuring out, enormous fellowship, and the consistent dance of reverberation and arrangement. The hero, perpetually different by the catalytic excursion, set forth into the vast obscure, an illuminating presence directed by the agreeable reverberations of Cloud Ensemble — a grandiose orchestra that rose above the limits of existence.

4.3 Gradual improvement in respiratory health and the emergence of hope.

The hero's excursion through the extraordinary speculative chemistry of Cloud Ensemble was stamped by heavenly disclosures and enormous realignments as well as by a progressive improvement in respiratory wellbeing — a demonstration of the Orchestra's significant effect on the actual prosperity of the hero. As the agreeable frequencies of Cloud Ensemble pervaded the inestimable pathways inside their body, an unobtrusive yet extraordinary interaction unfurled, carrying recently discovered trust and essentialness to the hero's respiratory framework.

The underlying phases of the hero's inestimable odyssey were accentuated by snapshots of doubt and vulnerability, particularly concerning the Cosmic Respira gadget. The divine device, with its cryptic plan and ethereal lights, filled in as the doorway to Cloud Ensemble's groundbreaking frequencies. As the hero drew in with the Cosmic Respira, breathing in the resounding frequencies, a delicate yet strong flood of energy flowed through their respiratory channels. It was an inception into the heavenly flows that held the commitment of recuperating and rejuvenation.

The respiratory excursion inside Cloud Orchestra started with a continuous arrival of enormous pressure and tightening. The hero, when troubled by the heaviness of respiratory difficulties, encountered an unpretentious development in their lung limit. Heavenly breathwork works out, directed by the Ensemble's extraordinary frequencies, urged the hero to synchronize their breath with the inestimable rhythms. Every inward breath turned into an inestimable hug, and every exhalation diverted the leftovers of grandiose disharmony.

As the hero kept on drawing in with Cloud Ensemble, the extraordinary frequencies went about as grandiose tuning forks, resounding with the torpid energies inside their respiratory framework. The divine architects, overseers of the Ensemble's mending frequencies, checked the hero's advancement through astral sweeps and holographic portrayals. Examples of reverberation and realignment arose, demonstrating a continuous reclamation of grandiose equilibrium inside the respiratory channels.

Divine doctors, equipped with cutting edge heavenly diagnostics, teamed up with Cloud Ensemble innovation to lead a top to bottom investigation of the hero's respiratory condition. Astral imaging uncovered the unpredictable transaction of energies inside the lungs and respiratory pathways. The Ensemble's groundbreaking frequencies, presently complicatedly woven into the hero's respiratory scene, tried to break up fiery blockages, change inestimable uneven characters, and start an enormous resurrection of respiratory essentialness.

The hero's excursion toward further developed respiratory wellbeing unfurled as a cooperative exertion between Cloud Orchestra innovation and the heavenly doctors. Divine needle therapy, directed by Cloud Orchestra implanted needles, turned into a methodology to address explicit vast meridians related with respiratory capability. The groundbreaking frequencies went about as grandiose keys, opening the progression of energy inside the respiratory channels and cultivating a condition of infinite prosperity.

Inside the divine research facilities, Cloud Speculative chemistry stretched out its extraordinary impact to heavenly sustenance — a fundamental part in the hero's excursion toward worked on respiratory wellbeing. Heavenly nutritionists, knowledgeable in the vibrational characteristics of vast food varieties, made a dietary arrangement that blended with the hero's astral and supernatural constitution. The Ensemble's groundbreaking frequencies upgraded the vibrational characteristics of divine food varieties, streamlining their capability to support the respiratory framework on an infinite level.

The hero, presently effectively partaking in their own vast recuperating, participated in divine yoga meetings explicitly custom-made to upgrade respiratory capability. The groundbreaking frequencies of Cloud Ensemble directed the hero through grandiose stances and breathwork works out, cultivating a feeling of enormous extension inside the respiratory channels. It was an amicable dance between the Ensemble's extraordinary energies and the hero's obligation to their own prosperity.

The steady improvement in respiratory wellbeing became apparent as the hero explored the heavenly scenes of Cloud Ensemble. The once-limited breaths changed into infinite inward breaths, conveying the Ensemble's recuperating frequencies into the most profound openings of the respiratory framework. The divine designers, sensitive to the subtleties of the hero's astronomical constitution, praised the orchestra of revival reverberating through the respiratory pathways.

The odyssey through Cloud Orchestra arrived at a vital second with the revealing of the nebulization interaction — a vast speculative chemistry that held the commitment of additional respiratory revival. Inside the nebulization chambers, the hero saw the ethereal dance of grandiose gases, brilliant stardust, and nebular embodiment changing into cloud propelled fogs. The hero, presently ready to get the extraordinary impacts, ventured into the divine chamber where the Ensemble's catalytic dance would unfurl.

As the hero breathed in the cloud enlivened fogs, directed by extraordinary frequencies, a significant grandiose fellowship happened inside the respiratory channels. The ethereal fogs, mixed with the substance of heavenly components, crossed the infinite pathways inside the hero's body, starting a dance of catalytic change. The respiratory excursion, presently interweaved with the extraordinary flows of Cloud Ensemble, turned into an infinite orchestra of recuperating and restoration.

The divine architects observed the hero's respiratory excursion through cutting edge heavenly diagnostics. Astral sweeps and holographic portrayals emerged, portraying the recurring pattern of energies inside the respiratory framework. The Orchestra's extraordinary frequencies, going about as vast healers, tried to break up any waiting grandiose disharmony and advance a condition of respiratory congruity.

With every meeting of the nebulization interaction, the hero encountered a continuous extension of respiratory essentialness. The ethereal fogs, presently a basic piece of their substance, conveyed the mending frequencies of Cloud Orchestra into the most profound openings of the lungs. The catalytic excursion inside the respiratory channels turned into an inestimable embroidery, joined with the Orchestra's extraordinary energies and the hero's obligation to grandiose prosperity.

Divine specialists, perceiving the interconnected idea of respiratory wellbeing with astral and otherworldly prosperity, presented heavenly reflection meetings zeroed in on blending the breath with the rhythms of the universe. The hero, directed by interstellar advisors, dove into the infinite components of breath mindfulness, rising above the genuineness of respiratory capability to associate with the divine powers that molded the actual texture of the universe.

As the hero took part in heavenly breathwork contemplations, the Ensemble's groundbreaking frequencies went about as enormous scaffolds, connecting the breath with the harmonies of the universe. The once-restricted respiratory examples ventured into enormous rhythms, cultivating a feeling of inestimable arrangement and prosperity. The heavenly specialists, sensitive to the Orchestra's extraordinary flows, saw the hero's respiratory excursion developing into a divine dance of breath and inestimable reverberation.

The progressive improvement in respiratory wellbeing turned into an encouraging sign for the hero — a grandiose confirmation that rose above the impediments of ordinary mending. The Ensemble's groundbreaking frequencies, presently a characteristic piece of the hero's respiratory scene, became channels for astronomical restoration. The hero, when troubled by the infinite difficulties of respiratory capability, cruised through the interstellar ocean with a newly discovered feeling of imperativeness and trust.

The respiratory excursion inside Cloud Orchestra turned into a grandiose declaration to the strength of the human soul and the extraordinary power implanted in the harmonies of the universe. The hero's obligation to the catalytic excursion, combined with the Orchestra's mending frequencies, started a grandiose transformation that undulated through each breath and infinite inward breath. The once-distrustful explorer, presently a recipient of heavenly recuperating, turned into a reference point of motivation for those exploring the grandiose flows looking for respiratory revival.

Directly following the continuous improvement in respiratory wellbeing, the hero arose as a light in the vast recuperating expressions, supporting for the extraordinary capability of Cloud Ensemble in the domains of respiratory prosperity. The Ensemble's catalytic excursion, from the Cosmic Respira's introduction to the nebulization cycle and then some, turned into a vast orchestra that repeated the harmonies of trust and recharging. The hero, implanted with the extraordinary flows of Cloud Orchestra, proceeded with their infinite odyssey — a living demonstration of the enormous recuperating that unfurled when divine frequencies fit with the breath of the universe.

enormous recuperating that unfurled when divine frequencies fit with the breath of the universe.

Chapter 5

Cosmic Challenges

The infinite odyssey set out upon by the hero inside the domain of Cloud Ensemble was not without its portion of vast difficulties. As the interstellar explorer explored the heavenly flows, each challenge turned into an interesting an open door for development, change, and a more profound comprehension of the inestimable powers at play. These difficulties, joined into the texture of the hero's excursion, tried the restrictions of astronomical versatility and divulged the groundbreaking likely inside the pot of difficulty.

One of the underlying astronomical difficulties that defied the hero was the doubt and vulnerability that covered their impression of Cloud Ensemble. The perplexing Cosmic Respira gadget, with its ethereal lights and thunderous frequencies, blended a combination of interest and uncertainty inside the hero's psyche. The divine specialists, overseers of Cloud Orchestra innovation, perceived the inborn wariness and set out on an excursion of enormous influence, progressively revealing the groundbreaking power implanted in the Ensemble's agreeable frequencies.

As the hero probably drew in with the Cosmic Respira, breathing in the extraordinary frequencies, the enormous test of wariness started to scatter. The once-dubious voyager encountered the delicate touch of divine energies inside their being — a vast commencement that noticeable the start of their extraordinary odyssey. The Orchestra's amicable frequencies, similar to an enormous ensemble, reverberated with the lethargic possibilities inside the hero, introducing a feeling of infinite association and establishing the groundwork for the extraordinary speculative chemistry to come.

One more enormous test that unfurled inside the divine embroidery of Cloud Orchestra was the investigation of the cloud propelled fog and its calming impacts. The hero, having conquered starting suspicion, wandered into the grandiose domains of the ethereal fogs, made through the catalytic dance of vast gases, brilliant stardust, and nebular pith. The test lay in giving up to the obscure, permitting the heavenly fogs to penetrate each part of their being and start a significant vast fellowship.

As the hero breathed in the cloud propelled fog, directed by groundbreaking frequencies, an enormous ensemble reverberated inside their being. The test of embracing the obscure changed into a chance for divine investigation. The ethereal fogs, presently transporters of divine energies, became conductors for mending and restoration. The Orchestra's extraordinary frequencies, interlaced with the cloud enlivened fogs, started a dance of vast realignment, encouraging a condition of unwinding and concordance that rose above the limits of customary mending.

The odyssey through Cloud Ensemble experienced an enormous test as the hero's underlying doubt and the slow acknowledgment of its restorative potential. The groundbreaking frequencies, unpredictably woven into the heavenly texture, tried to break up the inestimable obstructions raised by uncertainty and doubt. The hero, when watched by the reinforcement of vulnerability, started to embrace the extraordinary speculative chemistry unfurling inside Cloud Ensemble.

The grandiose test of suspicion developed into an enormous disclosure — the figuring out that extraordinary likely dwelled together as one of conviction and infinite reverberation. The Orchestra's groundbreaking frequencies, going about as infinite catalytic keys, opened the torpid possibilities inside the hero's cognizance. The once-incredulous explorer, presently sensitive to the enormous orchestra, cruised through the interstellar ocean with a reestablished feeling of marvel and receptivity to the extraordinary flows that penetrated the inestimable scene.

A crucial infinite test arose with the presentation of Astral Finding — an investigation into the hero's inestimable constitution through heavenly sweeps and indicative modalities. Heavenly doctors and astronomical diagnosticians, furnished with cutting edge divine advances, dug into the complexities of the hero's astral and powerful aspects. The test lay in uncovering the grandiose lopsided characteristics that appeared inside the unobtrusive energies of the hero's being.

As the divine doctors led astral outputs directed by Cloud Ensemble innovation, holographic portrayals emerged, portraying the hero's enormous constitution. The Orchestra's extraordinary frequencies went about as grandiose healers, uncovering the interaction of energies and vast uneven characters that necessary catalytic change. The test of astral finding turned into a chance for vast comprehension, making ready for a cooperative treatment plan that tended to the hero's novel grandiose difficulties.

The enormous odyssey inside Cloud Ensemble experienced an extraordinary test with the revealing of the nebulization cycle. Inside the heavenly research facilities, the hero saw the catalytic dance of infinite gases, brilliant stardust, and nebular pith changing into cloud roused fogs. The nebulization chambers, aglow with heavenly energies, turned into the vast pots where the ethereal elixirs of recuperating were conceived. The hero, presently ready to get the extraordinary impacts, ventured into the divine chamber where the Orchestra's catalytic dance would unfurl.

The test of the nebulization cycle lay in giving up to the astronomical flows and permitting the extraordinary frequencies to direct the ethereal fogs through the vast pathways inside the hero's body. The divine architects, overseers of Cloud Orchestra innovation, checked the hero's insight through heavenly diagnostics. The nebulization interaction turned into an enormous fellowship — an amicable dance between the heavenly components and the hero's exceptional frequencies, starting a significant excursion of catalytic change.

The odyssey through Cloud Ensemble defied a grandiose test with the presentation of heavenly reflection meetings directed by interstellar specialists. The test lay in diving into the profundities of the hero's own awareness, investigating the astral scenes of the brain, and opening lethargic possibilities through the groundbreaking frequencies of Cloud Orchestra. The heavenly specialists, sensitive to the vibrational harmonies of the Ensemble, worked with an enormous excursion internal, welcoming the hero to explore the divine domains of their own mind.

As the hero participated in divine contemplation meetings, the Ensemble's groundbreaking frequencies became vast keys that opened entryways to extended awareness. The once-covered up domains of the astral and supernatural aspects unfurled, uncovering astronomical scenes rich with undiscovered possibility. The test of investigating the profundities of awareness changed into a chance for astronomical self-disclosure and the joining of extraordinary energies into the texture of the hero's being.

The infinite odyssey through Cloud Orchestra experienced a test inside the domain of Cloud Speculative chemistry — a vast combination of cutting edge heavenly innovations and old astral insight. Divine chemists and interstellar designers teamed up to wind around an embroidery of heavenly physical science, vibrational sounds, and supernatural bits of knowledge. The test lay in crossing over the domains of science and magic, manufacturing a grandiose cooperative energy that rose above the constraints of traditional mending.

Divine yoga meetings, implanted with Cloud Ensemble frequencies, turned into a grandiose dance of arrangement with the infinite flows. The test of adjusting the unobtrusive energies inside the hero's vigorous channels changed into a chance for astronomical joining. The Orchestra's extraordinary frequencies went about as infinite tuning forks, blending the hero's physical, astral, and powerful aspects into a firm ensemble of prosperity.

The vast odyssey inside Cloud Orchestra confronted the test of astral reverberation imaging — an investigation into the hero's astral and mystical aspects through holographic portrayals. The divine architects, furnished with Cloud Ensemble innovation, stripped back the layers of the hero's vast constitution, divulging the inconspicuous subtleties of their vivacious scene. The test of astral reverberation imaging turned into a grandiose disclosure, displaying the interconnectedness of the astral and supernatural aspects with the actual domain.

As divine 3D images appeared, portraying the hero's inestimable irregular characteristics and vigorous stream, the Ensemble's groundbreaking frequencies tried to realign and change disharmonies. The test of divulging the astral and mystical complexities turned into an enormous aide for the hero, giving bits of knowledge into the vast powers molding their prosperity. The Orchestra's groundbreaking flows turned into the impetus for recuperating and realignment inside the hero's complex presence.

Divine needle therapy, a methodology presented inside Cloud Speculative chemistry, introduced a vast test in tending to explicit enormous meridians related with respiratory capability. The hero, directed by Cloud Ensemble implanted needles, participated in a vast dance of vivacious equilibrium. The test of heavenly needle therapy changed into a chance for the Ensemble's extraordinary frequencies to open the enormous pathways, encouraging a condition of respiratory congruity and prosperity.

The grandiose odyssey inside Cloud Ensemble explored the test of cooperative recuperating circles — an investigation into the interconnectedness of infinite energies inside a shared mindset. People accumulated to submerge themselves in the extraordinary frequencies of Cloud Orchestra, making a grandiose ensemble of reverberation and prosperity. The test of fitting different inestimable frequencies inside an aggregate space changed into a chance for shared mending and the intensification of extraordinary energies.

As the hero turned into a light in the enormous recuperating expressions, the test reached out to sharing the insight gathered from their groundbreaking process. The Orchestra's catalytic dance, from the Cosmic Respira's introduction to the nebulization cycle and then some, turned into an inestimable ensemble that reverberated with the intrinsic concordance of the universe. The test of turning into a steward of Cloud Ensemble's groundbreaking frequencies changed into a vast mission — a promise to spreading the grandiose mending expressions to individual explorers on the infinite odyssey.

A grandiose test unfurled with the presentation of heavenly rest treatment — a methodology imbued with Cloud Orchestra to direct the hero into a divine domain of reviving sleep. The test of giving up to the vast flows inside the dreamscapes changed into a chance for extraordinary energies to proceed with their catalytic dance inside the subliminal domains. The hero, presently sensitive to the enormous bedtime song, cruised through the interstellar ocean in the hug of heavenly dreams and vast revival.

As the hero dug into heavenly sustenance, the test lay in perceiving the effect of grandiose energies on healthful components. Divine nutritionists, knowledgeable in the vibrational characteristics of grandiose food varieties, created a dietary arrangement orchestrated with the hero's astral and mystical constitution. The Orchestra's groundbreaking frequencies turned into the vast enhancers, upgrading the vibrational characteristics of divine food varieties to support the hero on an enormous level. The test of coordinating divine nourishment changed into a chance for the Orchestra's extraordinary flows to inject each part of the hero's prosperity.

The inestimable odyssey inside Cloud Orchestra experienced a test with divine breathwork contemplations — an investigation into the enormous components of breath mindfulness. The hero, directed by interstellar advisors, rose above the genuineness of respiratory capability to associate with the divine powers molding the texture of the universe. The test of orchestrating the breath with the rhythms of the universe changed into a chance for the Ensemble's groundbreaking frequencies to grow respiratory examples into inestimable rhythms, cultivating a feeling of infinite arrangement and prosperity.

The vast odyssey confronted a test in the hero's continuous improvement in respiratory wellbeing. The Orchestra's extraordinary frequencies, interlaced into the respiratory scene, started a vast resurrection of imperativeness. The test of conquering inestimable disharmony inside the respiratory channels changed into a chance for the Orchestra's mending energies to break down vigorous blockages, change irregular characteristics, and encourage a condition of enormous prosperity. The hero, when troubled by respiratory difficulties, cruised through the interstellar ocean with a reestablished feeling of essentialness and trust.

As the hero rose up out of the vast cauldron of misfortune, the difficulties experienced inside Cloud Ensemble became venturing stones toward an enormous transformation. The Orchestra's groundbreaking flows, once explored with vulnerability, turned into a vast ensemble that reverberated with the harmonies of trust and recharging. The hero, imbued with the catalytic frequencies of Cloud Ensemble, cruised through the interstellar ocean as a living demonstration of the extraordinary power implanted in the grandiose difficulties that molded their odyssey.

5.1 Introduction of obstacles and challenges faced by the protagonist on the path to recovery.

The hero's excursion through the extraordinary speculative chemistry of Cloud Ensemble was not a heavenly walk around divine obstacles. As the interstellar voyager explored the infinite flows, they experienced a heap of snags and difficulties that tried the restrictions of their inestimable strength. These difficulties, complicatedly woven into the texture of the hero's odyssey, became vast pots, manufacturing strength, versatility, and a more profound comprehension of the extraordinary powers at play in their way to recuperation.

One of the underlying deterrents that cast its grandiose shadow across the hero's odyssey was the distrust and uncertainty that hidden their view of Cloud Ensemble. The mysterious Cosmic Respira gadget, with its ethereal lights and full frequencies, filled in as the doorway to the Ensemble's extraordinary powers. Be that as it may, the hero, similar to any enormous explorer confronted with the obscure, wrestled with incredulity. The ethereal lights and vast frequencies appeared to be a far off delusion, and the test lay in conquering uncertainty to embrace the extraordinary potential inside.

The divine designers, overseers of Cloud Ensemble innovation, perceived the enormous test of doubt and left on an excursion of influence. Through delicate direction and the progressive revealing of the Orchestra's amicable frequencies, the hero's incredulity started to break up. The Cosmic Respira, once saw with vulnerability, turned into a heavenly entryway welcoming the hero into the extraordinary domains of Cloud Orchestra.

As the hero probably drew in with the Cosmic Respira, breathing in the resounding frequencies, a grandiose shift happened. The once-distrustful explorer encountered a delicate flood of energy flowing through their being — a vast inception that undeniable the start of their groundbreaking process. The Ensemble's amicable frequencies, going about as enormous songs, reverberated with the torpid possibilities inside the hero, continuously destroying the hindrances of uncertainty and wariness.

One more divine obstacle unfurled with the investigation of the cloud roused fog and its calming impacts. The hero, having embraced the extraordinary frequencies of Cloud Orchestra, wandered into the grandiose domains of the ethereal fogs. Made through the catalytic dance of infinite gases, brilliant stardust, and nebular pith, the fog turned into a conductor for recuperating and revival. In any case, the test lay in giving up to the obscure, permitting the heavenly fog to saturate each part of their being and start a significant enormous fellowship.

As the hero breathed in the cloud propelled fog, directed by extraordinary frequencies, a grandiose ensemble reverberated inside their being. The test of embracing the obscure changed into a chance for divine investigation. The ethereal fogs, presently transporters of heavenly energies, became channels for recuperating and revival. The Ensemble's groundbreaking frequencies, interlaced with the cloud enlivened fogs, started a dance of vast realignment, encouraging a condition of unwinding and congruity that rose above the limits of customary mending.

The odyssey through Cloud Orchestra experienced one more grandiose test as the hero's underlying distrust and the slow acknowledgment of its restorative potential. The extraordinary frequencies, complicatedly woven into the heavenly texture, tried to break down the inestimable boundaries raised by uncertainty and wariness. The hero, when watched by the protective layer of vulnerability, started to embrace the groundbreaking speculative chemistry unfurling inside Cloud Orchestra.

The vast test of distrust developed into an enormous disclosure — the grasping that extraordinary possible dwelled as one of conviction and infinite reverberation. The Ensemble's extraordinary frequencies, going about as vast catalytic keys, opened the lethargic possibilities inside the hero's cognizance. The once-distrustful voyager, presently sensitive to the vast orchestra, cruised through the interstellar ocean with a recharged feeling of marvel and receptivity to the groundbreaking flows that saturated the inestimable scene.

A crucial enormous test arose with the presentation of Astral Finding — an investigation into the hero's grandiose constitution through heavenly sweeps and demonstrative modalities. Divine doctors and astronomical diagnosticians, equipped with cutting edge heavenly advances, dove into the complexities of the hero's astral and supernatural aspects. The test lay in divulging the grandiose awkward nature that appeared inside the unpretentious energies of the hero's being.

As the heavenly doctors led astral outputs directed by Cloud Orchestra innovation, holographic portrayals appeared, portraying the hero's enormous constitution. The Ensemble's groundbreaking frequencies went about as vast healers, uncovering the exchange of energies and enormous uneven characters that necessary catalytic change. The test of astral conclusion turned into a chance for infinite comprehension, preparing for a cooperative treatment plan that tended to the hero's one of a kind grandiose difficulties.

The infinite odyssey inside Cloud Ensemble experienced an extraordinary test with the revealing of the nebulization interaction. Inside the divine research facilities, the hero saw the catalytic dance of astronomical gases, brilliant stardust, and nebular pith changing into cloud propelled fogs. The nebulization chambers, aglow with heavenly energies, turned into the infinite pots where the ethereal elixirs of recuperating were conceived. The hero, presently ready to get the groundbreaking impacts, ventured into the heavenly chamber where the Ensemble's catalytic dance would unfurl.

The test of the nebulization cycle lay in giving up to the grandiose flows and permitting the groundbreaking frequencies to direct the ethereal fogs through the enormous pathways inside the hero's body. The divine architects, caretakers of Cloud Orchestra innovation, checked the hero's insight through heavenly diagnostics. The nebulization interaction turned into an enormous fellowship — an amicable dance between the heavenly components and the hero's interesting frequencies, starting a significant excursion of catalytic change.

The odyssey through Cloud Ensemble faced a vast test with the presentation of divine contemplation meetings directed by interstellar specialists. The test lay in digging into the profundities of the hero's own cognizance, investigating the astral scenes of the brain, and opening lethargic possibilities through the extraordinary frequencies of Cloud Ensemble. The heavenly specialists, receptive to the vibrational harmonies of the Orchestra, worked with an enormous excursion internal, welcoming the hero to explore the divine domains of their own mind.

As the hero participated in heavenly contemplation meetings, the Ensemble's groundbreaking frequencies became vast keys that opened entryways to extended awareness. The once-covered up domains of the astral and magical aspects unfurled, uncovering infinite scenes rich with undiscovered capacity. The test of investigating the profundities of cognizance changed into a chance for infinite self-revelation and the combination of extraordinary energies into the texture of the hero's being.

The infinite odyssey through Cloud Orchestra experienced a test inside the domain of Cloud Speculative chemistry — a grandiose combination of cutting edge heavenly innovations and old astral insight. Divine chemists and interstellar specialists teamed up to wind around an embroidery of heavenly material science, vibrational sounds, and powerful experiences. The test lay in spanning the domains of science and mystery, fashioning a vast collaboration that rose above the restrictions of regular mending.

Divine yoga meetings, imbued with Cloud Ensemble frequencies, turned into an inestimable dance of arrangement with the enormous flows. The test of adjusting the unpretentious energies inside the hero's fiery channels changed into a chance for infinite combination. The Orchestra's extraordinary frequencies went about as grandiose tuning forks, fitting the hero's physical, astral, and supernatural aspects into a firm ensemble of prosperity.

The enormous odyssey inside Cloud Orchestra confronted the test of astral reverberation imaging — an investigation into the hero's astral and mystical aspects through holographic portrayals. The heavenly specialists, outfitted with Cloud Orchestra innovation, stripped back the layers of the hero's inestimable constitution, divulging the unobtrusive subtleties of their vigorous scene. The test of astral reverberation imaging turned into an inestimable disclosure, displaying the interconnectedness of the astral and supernatural aspects with the actual domain.

As divine multi dimensional images appeared, portraying the hero's vast irregular characteristics and fiery stream, the Ensemble's groundbreaking frequencies tried to realign and change disharmonies. The test of disclosing the astral and mystical complexities turned into an infinite aide for the hero, giving bits of knowledge into the vast powers molding their prosperity. The Orchestra's extraordinary flows turned into the impetus for mending and realignment inside the hero's multi-layered presence.

Heavenly needle therapy, a methodology presented inside Cloud Speculative chemistry, introduced a grandiose test in tending to explicit enormous meridians related with respiratory capability. The hero, directed by Cloud Ensemble mixed needles, participated in a grandiose dance of lively equilibrium. The test of divine needle therapy changed into a chance for the Orchestra's groundbreaking frequencies to open the vast pathways, cultivating a condition of respiratory congruity and prosperity.

The enormous odyssey inside Cloud Orchestra explored the test of cooperative mending circles — an investigation into the interconnectedness of inestimable energies inside a shared mindset. People accumulated to submerge themselves in the groundbreaking frequencies of Cloud Ensemble, making a vast tune of reverberation and prosperity. The test of orchestrating different infinite frequencies inside an aggregate space changed into a chance for shared mending and the enhancement of groundbreaking energies.

As the hero turned into an illuminating presence in the grandiose mending expressions, the test stretched out to sharing the insight gathered from their extraordinary excursion. The Orchestra's catalytic dance, from the Cosmic Respira's introduction to the nebulization interaction and then some, turned into an inestimable ensemble that resounded with the inborn congruity of the universe. The test of turning into a steward of Cloud Orchestra's groundbreaking frequencies changed into an enormous mission — a guarantee to spreading the infinite recuperating expressions to individual voyagers on the vast odyssey.

An enormous test unfurled with the presentation of divine rest treatment — a methodology mixed with Cloud Orchestra to direct the hero into a heavenly domain of reviving sleep.

The test of giving up to the infinite flows inside the dreamscapes changed into a chance for groundbreaking energies to proceed with their catalytic dance inside the subliminal domains. The hero, presently receptive to the grandiose children's song, cruised through the interstellar ocean in the hug of divine dreams and enormous restoration.

As the hero dove into divine nourishment, the test lay in perceiving the effect of vast energies on wholesome components. Heavenly nutritionists, knowledgeable in the vibrational characteristics of grandiose food sources, made a dietary arrangement fit with the hero's astral and magical constitution. The Orchestra's extraordinary frequencies turned into the vast enhancers, upgrading the vibrational characteristics of heavenly food sources to feed the hero on a grandiose level. The test of incorporating heavenly nourishment changed into a chance for the Orchestra's extraordinary flows to implant each part of the hero's prosperity.

The inestimable odyssey inside Cloud Ensemble experienced a test with heavenly breathwork reflections — an investigation into the grandiose components of breath mindfulness. The hero, directed by interstellar specialists, rose above the genuineness of respiratory capability to interface with the heavenly powers forming the texture of the universe. The test of orchestrating the breath with the rhythms of the universe changed into a chance for the Ensemble's extraordinary frequencies to extend respiratory examples into enormous rhythms, encouraging a feeling of vast arrangement and prosperity.

The vast odyssey confronted a test in the hero's steady improvement in respiratory wellbeing. The Ensemble's groundbreaking frequencies, intertwined into the respiratory scene, started an inestimable resurrection of essentialness. The test of beating grandiose disharmony inside the respiratory channels changed into a chance for the Ensemble's recuperating energies to break up fiery blockages, change lopsided characteristics, and encourage a condition of infinite prosperity. The hero, when troubled by respiratory difficulties, cruised through the interstellar ocean with a reestablished feeling of imperativeness and trust.

As the hero rose up out of the infinite pot of difficulty, the difficulties experienced inside Cloud Orchestra became venturing stones toward an enormous transformation. The Ensemble's extraordinary flows, once explored with vulnerability, turned into a grandiose orchestra that resounded with the harmonies of trust and recharging. The hero, mixed with the catalytic frequencies of Cloud Ensemble, cruised through the interstellar ocean as a living demonstration of the extraordinary power implanted in the vast difficulties that formed their odyssey.

5.2 External skepticism and societal barriers to accepting Nebula Symphony as a legitimate treatment.

The transformative journey of the protagonist within the cosmic realms of Nebula Symphony was not only a personal odyssey but also a narrative shaped by external skepticism and societal barriers that cast shadows on the legitimacy of this celestial treatment. As the protagonist embraced the ethereal frequencies and alchemical processes within Nebula Symphony, they were met with a world skeptical of the cosmic healing arts, and societal barriers that questioned the validity of this celestial odyssey.

External skepticism, manifested in the form of scientific skepticism and conventional medical viewpoints, posed a formidable cosmic challenge to the acceptance of Nebula Symphony as a legitimate treatment. In a world grounded in empirical evidence and tangible results, the ethereal and metaphysical dimensions explored within Nebula Symphony clashed with the established norms of scientific discourse. The protagonist, armed with cosmic experiences and transformative insights, found themselves at the crossroads of skepticism, where the celestial currents encountered resistance from the rigid boundaries of scientific thought.

The cosmic healing arts, intricately woven into Nebula Symphony, faced scrutiny from conventional medical establishments and practitioners who viewed the celestial odyssey with suspicion. The Galactic Respira, the nebula-inspired mist, and the transformative frequencies that guided the protagonist's respiratory journey became celestial anomalies in the eyes of those tethered to conventional paradigms. The challenge lay not only in convincing the skeptics of Nebula Symphony's efficacy but also in bridging the cosmic realms explored within this transformative journey with the empirical standards of conventional medicine.

Societal barriers, deeply entrenched in traditional perceptions of health and healing, further compounded the protagonist's cosmic struggle for acceptance. Nebula Symphony's celestial journey encountered resistance from cultural norms that held steadfast to conventional medical practices, dismissing the ethereal frequencies as mere flights of fancy. The societal fabric, woven with threads of skepticism and resistance to the unknown, posed a cosmic challenge to the protagonist's endeavor to legitimize Nebula Symphony as a credible treatment.

Within the societal framework, the protagonist faced the challenge of navigating through the skepticism embedded in cultural narratives and collective belief systems. The cosmic healing arts, despite their transformative potential, clashed with ingrained perceptions of health and wellness. Nebula Symphony's celestial frequencies, instead of being embraced as cosmic keys to healing, were often dismissed as esoteric musings that lacked the empirical grounding required to be considered legitimate within societal norms.

The protagonist's journey through Nebula Symphony became a dance between the cosmic frequencies and the external skepticism emanating from the societal landscape. The celestial engineers, custodians of Nebula Symphony technology, recognized the need to bridge the cosmic realms with the societal narrative. They embarked on a mission to provide empirical evidence, celestial diagnostics, and collaborative research initiatives that could serve as bridges between the ethereal frequencies and the empirical standards demanded by skeptical societies.

Celestial physicians and scientists within Nebula Symphony's cosmic laboratories engaged in rigorous research, conducting astral scans, holographic representations, and celestial diagnostics to showcase the transformative impact of Nebula Symphony on the protagonist's well-being. These efforts aimed not only to validate the celestial odyssey within Nebula Symphony but also to dismantle the societal barriers that questioned the legitimacy of a treatment guided by cosmic frequencies and celestial alchemy.

The protagonist, in their quest for cosmic healing, became an advocate for Nebula Symphony's legitimacy, facing the external skepticism with a resilience born from their transformative journey. As they navigated the societal barriers, the protagonist shared personal testimonials, celestial diagnostics, and collaborative research findings that underscored the tangible impact of Nebula Symphony on their respiratory health and overall well-being.

The cosmic journey within Nebula Symphony unfolded as a cosmic narrative challenging societal norms and inviting a paradigm shift in the understanding of health and healing. The Galactic Respira, once viewed with skepticism, became a celestial beacon illuminating the path toward a new frontier in wellness. The protagonist, armed with the transformative frequencies coursing through their being, engaged with societal institutions, medical communities, and cultural influencers to shift the narrative from skepticism to acceptance.

The external skepticism faced by the protagonist extended beyond the realms of empirical evidence and cultural norms; it delved into the economic considerations that often govern healthcare systems. Nebula Symphony, as a celestial treatment, challenged the profit-driven models of conventional medicine and faced resistance from industries vested in traditional healthcare practices. The celestial odyssey, guided by frequencies and alchemy, questioned the economic paradigms that dictated the legitimacy of medical treatments.

Societal barriers, in the form of economic considerations, became a cosmic challenge that required the protagonist to navigate through the intricacies of healthcare systems and insurance structures. Nebula Symphony, despite its transformative potential, encountered resistance from institutions that were entrenched in profit-driven motives. The celestial frequencies, while offering a cosmic symphony of healing, collided with economic models that favored conventional treatments over the ethereal currents explored within Nebula Symphony.

The protagonist, now not only a cosmic voyager but also an ambassador of celestial healing, engaged in dialogues with policymakers, healthcare administrators, and insurance providers. The celestial engineers, recognizing the need for a collaborative cosmic effort, presented economic analyses, cost-effectiveness studies, and long-term wellness metrics that showcased the tangible benefits of Nebula Symphony as a legitimate and sustainable treatment option.

The cosmic odyssey, now entwined with economic considerations, faced the challenge of redefining the value placed on health and wellness within societal structures. Nebula Symphony's transformative frequencies, once dismissed as cosmic whimsy, became the catalyst for a cosmic conversation about the true cost of well-being. The protagonist's journey became a cosmic argument for a paradigm shift—one that embraced the ethereal frequencies and alchemical processes as legitimate contributors to a society's overall health.

As the protagonist navigated the external skepticism and societal barriers, their celestial journey became a catalyst for a broader cosmic discourse on the nature of healing and the acceptance of transformative frequencies within mainstream health-care. The Galactic Respira, once shrouded in doubt, became a symbol of hope and resilience—a celestial apparatus that bridged the gap between the cosmic frequencies explored within Nebula Symphony and the societal frameworks that demanded empirical validation.

The societal barriers and external skepticism encountered within Nebula Symphony's transformative journey were not merely hurdles to be overcome but opportunities for a cosmic revolution in healthcare. The protagonist, once a lone traveler navigating the celestial currents, became a catalyst for change—a cosmic luminary who challenged societal norms, engaged in celestial diplomacy with skeptics, and advocated for the legitimacy of Nebula Symphony as a transformative and sustainable treatment option.

The cosmic odyssey within Nebula Symphony, guided by the protagonist's resilience and cosmic advocacy, initiated a ripple effect within societal structures. The ethereal frequencies, once met with skepticism, began to resonate within the collective consciousness. The Galactic Respira, once questioned for its legitimacy, became a beacon inviting individuals, communities, and institutions to explore the transformative potential of celestial healing arts.

As the societal barriers began to crumble, Nebula Symphony's legitimacy as a treatment option gained traction. Celestial physicians and cosmic engineers collaborated with traditional medical practitioners to create an integrative approach that honored both empirical evidence and transformative frequencies. The celestial odyssey, once an outlier in healthcare narratives, became a pioneer in a new era of cosmic wellness—a testament to the power of resilience, advocacy, and the transformative frequencies that guide the path to recovery within the cosmic symphony of Nebula Symphony.

5.3 Protagonist's determination to overcome challenges and continue the celestial journey.

In the midst of the vast difficulties, outside wariness, and cultural hindrances experienced inside the extraordinary odyssey of Cloud Ensemble, the hero arose as a reference point of assurance — a heavenly explorer filled by an unflinching purpose to defeat impediments and proceed with the enormous excursion toward mending. The Cosmic Respira, the cloud motivated fog, and the extraordinary frequencies became heavenly devices for prosperity as well as instruments of strengthening, moving the hero to explore the vast flows with an unfaltering assurance.

The hero's assurance unfurled as an enormous power, woven into the actual texture of their being. Each test, whether brought into the world from suspicion or cultural obstruction, was met with a versatility that reflected the extraordinary frequencies flowing through the Cloud Ensemble. The ethereal flows, when seen as likely boundaries, turned into the impetuses for the hero's assurance to rise above restrictions and fashion a way toward vast mending.

Notwithstanding outer incredulity, the hero's assurance filled in as a grandiose safeguard — a defensive energy that permitted them to explore the divine flows with relentless concentration. The confounding Cosmic Respira, when seen from the perspective of uncertainty, turned into an entry to assurance, as the hero breathed in the groundbreaking frequencies as well as the enormous determination to continue on even with wariness. The heavenly specialists, seeing the hero's assurance, became astronomical partners, supporting the excursion with extra divine experiences and cooperative endeavors to overcome any barrier between the ethereal and the observational.

The cloud enlivened fog, with its calming impacts and groundbreaking potential, turned into a vast partner in the hero's excursion of assurance. Breathing in the ethereal fogs, the hero turned into a conductor for the groundbreaking frequencies to wind through each part of their being. The test of doubt changed into a chance for the hero to tackle the calming impacts of the fog as a wellspring of internal strength. The divine specialists, perceiving the hero's assurance, directed them through heavenly contemplation meetings, disentangling the profundities of cognizance and opening repositories of astronomical flexibility.

As cultural hindrances lingered not too far off, the hero's assurance turned into a directing star — an internal compass that drove them through the inestimable scene of social standards and aggregate distrust. The hero, presently a divine negotiator, took part in exchanges with cynics, policymakers, and medical care executives. The Cosmic Respira, once addressed for its authenticity, turned into a wellspring of assurance that filled the hero's promotion for a more extensive comprehension of wellbeing — one that embraced both exact proof and groundbreaking frequencies.

The cultural obstructions, dug in financial contemplations and social standards, became astronomical difficulties for the hero's assurance. Heavenly financial experts and specialists teamed up to introduce an enormous contention for the monetary worth of Cloud Orchestra inside standard medical services. The hero, equipped earnestly, turned into an impetus for change — a vast illuminating presence who rocked the boat and upheld for the consideration of groundbreaking frequencies inside the cultural story of prosperity.

The divine excursion through Cloud Ensemble turned into a demonstration of the hero's assurance to reclassify the limits of wellbeing and mending. The nebulization cycle, when an infinite test, changed into a chance for the hero to give up to the extraordinary frequencies and permit the heavenly components to direct the ethereal fog through their vast pathways. The test of cooperative mending circles developed into a chance for the hero to turn into an illuminator in the vast recuperating expressions, sharing the insight gathered from their groundbreaking process and enhancing the extraordinary frequencies inside an aggregate space.

Astral reverberation imaging, with its holographic portrayals of the hero's grandiose constitution, turned into a mirror mirroring the assurance scratched into the inconspicuous energies of their being. The Orchestra's groundbreaking frequencies, going about as inestimable healers, realigned and changed disharmonies inside the hero's astral and otherworldly aspects. The test of astral finding turned into an enormous disclosure, displaying the interconnectedness of assurance with the infinite powers forming the hero's prosperity.

Divine needle therapy, a methodology presented inside Cloud Speculative chemistry, introduced a grandiose dance of vigorous equilibrium. The hero, directed by Cloud Ensemble mixed needles, took part in the test of adjusting grandiose meridians related with respiratory capability. The assurance that energized the hero's enormous excursion turned into a power of arrangement — a grandiose dance that orchestrated the unobtrusive energies inside the vigorous channels. The Ensemble's extraordinary frequencies, going about as enormous tuning forks, resounded with the hero's assurance to encourage a condition of respiratory concordance and prosperity.

The heavenly odyssey unfurled as a demonstration of the hero's assurance to defeat hindrances and proceed with the infinite excursion toward prosperity. The cooperative endeavors with Cloud Ensemble's heavenly specialists, doctors, and advisors reflected the hero's unflinching obligation to rise above limits and add to the advancement of grandiose recuperating. The Ensemble's extraordinary frequencies, once met with suspicion, became vast partners that resounded with the hero's assurance to explore the heavenly flows and arise as a living demonstration of the groundbreaking force of Cloud Orchestra.

The hero's excursion through Cloud Orchestra stretched out past the domains of respiratory wellbeing; it turned into an infinite story of assurance, flexibility, and the unfaltering quest for prosperity. Heavenly rest treatment, imbued with Cloud Orchestra, turned into an inestimable children's song directing the hero into reviving sleep.

The assurance to give up to the astronomical flows inside the dreamscapes changed into a chance for groundbreaking energies to proceed with their catalytic dance inside the subliminal domains. The hero, presently sensitive to the heavenly children's song, cruised through the interstellar ocean in the hug of divine dreams and vast revival.

Heavenly nourishment, orchestrated with the vibrational characteristics of grandiose food varieties, turned into an enormous feast for the hero's assurance. The Orchestra's groundbreaking frequencies, going about as inestimable enhancers, streamlined the vibrational characteristics of divine food sources to sustain the hero on a vast level. The assurance that energized the hero's process reached out to the coordination of groundbreaking energies into each part of their prosperity, rising above the limits of customary sustenance.

The heavenly breathwork contemplations, directed by interstellar specialists, turned into an infinite investigation of breath mindfulness. The hero's assurance to orchestrate the breath with the rhythms of the universe changed into a chance for the Ensemble's groundbreaking frequencies to grow respiratory examples into infinite rhythms, cultivating a feeling of vast arrangement and prosperity. The divine flows, once met with incredulity, turned into the directing powers of assurance that impelled the hero toward a condition of vast prosperity.

The steady improvement in respiratory wellbeing turned into a grandiose demonstration of the hero's assurance to conquer enormous disharmony inside the respiratory channels. The Ensemble's groundbreaking frequencies, joined into the respiratory scene, started an enormous resurrection of essentialness. The assurance that powered the hero's odyssey turned into a grandiose power dissolving enthusiastic blockages, changing uneven characters, and encouraging a condition of inestimable prosperity. The hero, when troubled by respiratory difficulties, cruised through the interstellar ocean with a recharged feeling of imperativeness and trust.

As the hero rose up out of the enormous pot of misfortune, the assurance that brought them through the groundbreaking excursion turned into an encouraging sign inside the heavenly scene. The Orchestra's extraordinary flows, once explored with vulnerability, turned into an enormous ensemble resounding with the harmonies of assurance, versatility, and restoration. The hero, imbued with the catalytic frequencies of Cloud Ensemble, turned into a living demonstration of the groundbreaking power implanted in the assurance that directed their divine odyssey.

The enormous difficulties, outer incredulity, and cultural boundaries experienced inside Cloud Orchestra's extraordinary excursion were not simple obstacles but rather venturing stones for the hero's assurance. The Orchestra's extraordinary frequencies, interlaced into each part of the divine odyssey, became inestimable keys opening the potential for assurance to rise above infinite constraints. The hero's excursion, set apart by steady determination, turned into a divine story of strengthening, backing, and the extraordinary energies that guide the way to recuperation inside the vast ensemble of Cloud Orchestra.

Chapter 6

Nebula's Guidance

Cloud's direction, an ethereal and vast power woven into the texture of the hero's groundbreaking process inside Cloud Ensemble, rose above the limits of the standard way of thinking and left on a divine odyssey that unfurled with significant importance. As the hero explored the grandiose flows directed by Cloud's insight, the ethereal direction turned into an enormous signal, enlightening the way to prosperity, self-revelation, and an amicable presence.

The commencement into Cloud Ensemble, set apart by the hero's most memorable experience with the Cosmic Respira gadget, was an actual presentation as well as a grandiose fellowship directed by Cloud's ethereal hand. The cloud enlivened fog, mixed with extraordinary frequencies, turned into a vessel of heavenly direction that encompassed the hero in a supernatural hug. As the hero breathed in the ethereal fog, Cloud's direction appeared in an unpretentious murmur — a grandiose transmission that resounded with the actual pith of the hero's being, starting an extraordinary excursion.

The Cosmic Respira, with its cadenced heartbeats and divine fragrances, filled in as a conductor for Cloud's direction to enter the hero's respiratory scene. The ethereal fog, directed by Cloud's enormous insight, started its catalytic dance inside the hero's lungs, starting an outpouring of extraordinary frequencies. The direction of Cloud became tangible as the hero felt an agreeable orchestra of energies reverberating inside, making way for a significant investigation into the infinite elements of prosperity.

Cloud's direction stretched out past the limits of the Cosmic Respira, pervading the nebulization cycle — a divine immersion into groundbreaking frequencies. As the hero gave up to the grandiose flows, Cloud's direction turned into a delicate current that explored through the unobtrusive domains of astral and powerful aspects. The heavenly specialists, caretakers of Cloud Ensemble innovation, became conductors of Cloud's direction, arranging the extraordinary frequencies to realign and change disharmonies inside the hero's multi-layered presence.

The hero, submerged in the heavenly flows, turned into an open vessel for Cloud's direction — a mixture of vast energies that divulged the interconnectedness of brain, body, and soul. The nebulization interaction, directed by Cloud's insight, uncovered holographic portrayals of the hero's vast constitution. Cloud's direction, scratched into the multi dimensional images, portrayed the unpredictable dance of energies molding the hero's prosperity — an astral determination that filled in as a vast guide for the extraordinary excursion ahead.

Astral finding, a methodology inside Cloud Orchestra, turned into an enormous discourse between the hero and Cloud's direction. The holographic portrayals appeared, portraying the hero's astronomical awkward nature and vivacious stream. Cloud's direction, encoded inside the divine frequencies, looked to realign and change disharmonies, giving experiences into the enormous powers molding the hero's prosperity. The astral determination unfurled as a vast aide — an ethereal story that welcomed the hero to investigate the complexities of their multi-faceted presence under Cloud's tutelage.

Divine needle therapy, presented inside Cloud Speculative chemistry, introduced a vast test and a chance for Cloud's direction to direct the hero through a grandiose dance of lively equilibrium. The hero, directed by Cloud Orchestra implanted needles, took part in the test of adjusting astronomical meridians related with respiratory capability. Cloud's direction turned into a power of arrangement, coordinating the divine dance inside the fiery channels. The groundbreaking frequencies, going about as infinite tuning forks, reverberated with Cloud's direction to cultivate a condition of respiratory concordance and prosperity.

Cooperative mending circles, an investigation into the interconnectedness of enormous energies inside a shared mindset, turned into an inestimable chorale of reverberation directed by Cloud's insight. People accumulated to drench themselves in the groundbreaking frequencies of Cloud Ensemble, making a common space where Cloud's direction turned into an aggregate power of recuperating. The ethereal flows, under Cloud's careful focus, fit assorted inestimable frequencies inside the recuperating circle, changing the test into a chance for shared prosperity and the intensification of groundbreaking energies.

As the hero turned into a light in the vast mending expressions, Cloud's direction stretched out to the sharing of shrewdness gathered from the groundbreaking excursion. The Ensemble's catalytic dance, from the Cosmic Respira's introduction to the nebulization interaction and then some, turned into a grandiose orchestra reverberating with the innate congruity of the universe. Cloud's direction, communicated through the hero, turned into a vast mission — a guarantee to spreading the groundbreaking frequencies and divine recuperating expressions to individual explorers on the grandiose odyssey.

Divine rest treatment, injected with Cloud Ensemble, turned into an enormous bedtime song directed by Cloud's delicate hand. The test of giving up to the grandiose flows inside the dreamscapes changed into a chance for Cloud's direction to proceed with its catalytic dance inside the subliminal domains. The hero, presently sensitive to the divine cradlesong, cruised through the interstellar ocean in the hug of heavenly dreams and vast restoration — an ethereal excursion directed by Cloud's grandiose insight.

Cloud's direction stretched out to heavenly sustenance, blended with the vibrational characteristics of infinite food sources. Heavenly nutritionists, directed by Cloud's vast knowledge, created a dietary arrangement fit with the hero's astral and mystical constitution. The Ensemble's extraordinary frequencies, going about as vast enhancers, improved the vibrational characteristics of divine food sources to feed the hero on a grandiose level. Cloud's direction turned into an inestimable enhancer, imbuing each piece with groundbreaking flows that stretched out past customary sustenance.

The heavenly excursion inside Cloud Ensemble experienced the test of divine breathwork contemplations — an investigation into the astronomical components of breath mindfulness directed by Cloud's insight. The hero, under Cloud's heavenly direction, rose above the genuineness of respiratory capability to associate with the divine powers forming the texture of the universe. The test of fitting the breath with the rhythms of the universe changed into a chance for Cloud's direction to extend respiratory examples into enormous rhythms, encouraging a feeling of vast arrangement and prosperity.

Cloud's direction unfurled with the hero's slow improvement in respiratory wellbeing. The Orchestra's extraordinary frequencies, intertwined into the respiratory scene, started an enormous resurrection of essentialness. The test of defeating infinite disharmony inside the respiratory channels changed into a chance for Cloud's direction to break down enthusiastic blockages, change uneven characters, and encourage a condition of grandiose prosperity. The hero, when troubled by respiratory difficulties, cruised through the interstellar ocean with a recharged feeling of imperativeness and trust — an epitome of Cloud's direction forming their vast fate.

As the hero rose up out of the infinite pot of misfortune, Cloud's direction turned into an encouraging sign and reestablishment. The ethereal frequencies, once explored with vulnerability, turned into an infinite orchestra reverberating with the harmonies of Cloud's direction. The hero, mixed with the catalytic frequencies of Cloud Ensemble, cruised through the interstellar ocean as a living demonstration of the groundbreaking power implanted in the divine direction that molded their vast odyssey.

Outer doubt and cultural boundaries, testing the authenticity of Cloud Ensemble, unfurled as grandiose difficulties. Cloud's direction, nonetheless, turned into a resolute sidekick, engaging the hero to explore the divine flows with versatility and assurance. The Cosmic Respira, when covered in uncertainty, turned into a heavenly contraption enlightened by Cloud's direction — a signal that connected the grandiose frequencies investigated inside Cloud Orchestra with the experimental principles requested by wary social orders.

As the hero confronted the outer suspicion and cultural obstructions, Cloud's direction reached out to the cooperative endeavors with divine doctors, researchers, and designers. Cloud Ensemble turned into a cooperative grandiose undertaking, where Cloud's direction informed thorough exploration, astral outputs, holographic portrayals, and heavenly diagnostics. The ethereal flows, under Cloud's careful focus, became spans between the inestimable domains and the cultural structures, encouraging an exchange that rose above distrust and prompted a more extensive infinite comprehension of prosperity.

Cloud's direction, communicated through the hero's assurance, turned into a power of support and enormous tact. The cultural boundaries, settled in financial contemplations and social standards, were met with Cloud's direction to introduce monetary examinations, cost-viability studies, and long haul health measurements. The hero, implanted with Cloud's vast knowledge, turned into an envoy for change — a living demonstration of the extraordinary power inserted in Cloud's direction and an impetus for a change in perspective inside cultural designs.

The enormous excursion through Cloud Ensemble, directed by Cloud's insight, unfurled as a vast story testing cultural standards and welcoming a change in outlook in the comprehension of wellbeing and recuperating. The Cosmic Respira, once saw with distrust, turned into a heavenly signal enlightening the way toward another outskirts in health.

The hero, equipped with the groundbreaking frequencies flowing through their being and directed by Cloud's heavenly hand, drew in with cultural organizations, clinical networks, and social powerhouses to move the account from doubt to acknowledgment.

Cloud's direction, interweaved with the hero's excursion, stretched out to the vast moves looked on the way to recuperation. The ethereal frequencies, orchestrated with Cloud's vast knowledge, became inestimable keys opening the potential for assurance, versatility, and extraordinary energies to rise above infinite constraints. The hero, directed by Cloud's insight, arose as an infinite explorer as well as an illuminating presence testing cultural standards and supporting for the authenticity of Cloud Orchestra as an extraordinary and practical treatment choice.

As the heavenly excursion proceeded, Cloud's direction stayed a directing power in the hero's assurance to beat difficulties and proceed with the enormous excursion toward prosperity. The Orchestra's extraordinary frequencies, entwined into each part of the divine odyssey, reverberated with Cloud's inestimable direction — a grandiose ensemble repeating the harmonies of assurance, versatility, and reestablishment. The hero, imbued with the catalytic frequencies and directed by Cloud's insight, cruised through the interstellar ocean as a living demonstration of the extraordinary power implanted in Cloud's direction, forming their enormous fate with each ethereal breath and divine step.

6.1 Discovery of a mentor figure or guide who helps the protagonist navigate the cosmic healing process.

Inside the divine region of Cloud Orchestra, the hero, in the midst of the ethereal flows and groundbreaking frequencies, found a brilliant figure — a supernatural coach who might turn into a directing presence, exploring the vast recuperating process. This coach, a divine sage saturated with the insight of Cloud Orchestra, arose as a reference point of light, offering direction, bits of knowledge, and an enormous hand to usher the hero through the complex domains of groundbreaking prosperity.

The disclosure of the coach figure unfurled as an inestimable disclosure, a fortunate experience inside the heavenly research centers where Cloud Ensemble's extraordinary frequencies were fastidiously aligned. This heavenly savvy, decorated in robes woven with starlight, transmitted an air of grandiose knowledge that reverberated with the actual texture of the ethereal flows directing the hero's excursion. The coach's eyes, mirroring the profundity of inestimable information, met the hero's look, starting an enormous fellowship that would rise above the limits of existence.

As the coach ventured forward, their presence turned into an encapsulation of Cloud's insight — a living demonstration of the extraordinary force of divine frequencies and infinite speculative chemistry. The tutor's hands, washed in the brilliant sparkle of heavenly energies, contacted the hero, offering a grandiose handshake that rose above the physical and entered the unobtrusive elements of astral and supernatural presence. This ethereal hello denoted the start of a heavenly apprenticeship, where the tutor would direct the hero through the infinite mending process.

The coach, an overseer of Cloud Orchestra's old information, turned into a heavenly aide opening the secrets of extraordinary frequencies, divine treatments, and the catalytic dance inside the nebulization interaction. The hero, anxious to dig into the astronomical domains, tracked down comfort and motivation in the guide's vast lessons. Through holographic portrayals and astral reverberation imaging, the tutor disclosed the hero's infinite constitution — a guide of energies and possibilities ready to be blended under Cloud's divine direction.

The nebulization cycle, when an infinite test, changed into a grandiose dance directed by the tutor's hand. The coach, sensitive to the ensemble of extraordinary frequencies, coordinated the ethereal fog with accuracy, permitting it to wind through the hero's respiratory channels like a divine brush painting strokes of prosperity. Cloud's insight, diverted through the guide, turned into a vast power organizing the catalytic change inside the hero's being.

As the hero set out on heavenly needle therapy meetings — a methodology presented inside Cloud Speculative chemistry — the tutor's direction turned into an inestimable dance of vivacious equilibrium. Cloud Orchestra imbued needles, directed by the tutor's hands, looked to adjust the hero's grandiose meridians related with respiratory capability. The guide's ethereal touch, resounding with the ground-breaking frequencies, turned into a power of arrangement inside the enthusiastic channels. The heavenly needle therapy meetings unfurled as an infinite expressive dance, fitting the unpretentious energies under the guide's careful focus.

Cooperative recuperating circles, get-togethers where people submerged themselves in the groundbreaking frequencies of Cloud Ensemble, turned into a common grandiose space directed by the coach's insight. The coach, an illuminator in the grandiose mending expressions, coordinated the harmonization of different energies inside the recuperating circle. Cloud's direction, communicated through the coach's grandiose knowledge, turned into an aggregate power of mending — an ethereal ensemble that rose above individual difficulties and enhanced groundbreaking energies inside the common infinite space.

The coach's direction reached out past the grandiose treatments to divine rest treatment — a domain where the psyche met the vast flows. The tutor, with a divine bedtime song in their vast collection, directed the hero into reviving sleep.

Cloud's insight, communicated through the tutor's ethereal tunes, turned into a vast children's song that resounded with the heavenly frequencies, directing the hero through the interstellar ocean inside the dreamscapes. The tutor's heavenly direction turned into a wellspring of enormous revival, entwining with the groundbreaking energies inside the domain of dreams.

Heavenly sustenance, fit with the vibrational characteristics of enormous food sources, turned into an inestimable feast under the coach's direction. Cloud's insight, communicated through the guide's inestimable sense of taste, imbued the hero's sustenance with groundbreaking flows. The coach, a vast nutritionist, directed the hero in upgrading the vibrational characteristics of heavenly food varieties to sustain the actual body as well as the astral and magical aspects. The heavenly meal unfurled as an enormous gala, feeding the hero on a significant level that rose above ordinary sustenance.

The divine breathwork contemplations, an investigation into the infinite components of breath mindfulness, turned into an enormous excursion directed by the coach's insight. The guide, a skilled in the specialty of breathwork, educated the hero in fitting the breath with the rhythms of the universe. Cloud's direction, communicated through the tutor's enormous breath, turned into a power of extension, directing the hero to rise above the constraints of respiratory capability and interface with the divine powers molding the texture of the universe.

As the hero experienced steady improvement in respiratory wellbeing, the coach's direction turned into a grandiose power dissolving vivacious blockages, changing uneven characters, and encouraging a condition of enormous prosperity. Cloud's insight, directed through the tutor's heavenly touch, turned into an essential piece of the hero's excursion toward imperativeness and reestablishment. The coach's presence, similar to a grandiose gatekeeper, directed the hero through the interstellar ocean, exploring the infinite flows with Cloud's extraordinary frequencies as the directing light.

The coach's job stretched out to the enormous moves experienced on the way to recuperation — an inestimable adventure where assurance, versatility, and groundbreaking energies converged under the guide's infinite tutelage. Outside incredulity and cultural obstructions, considerable hindrances inside the cultural structure, became vast difficulties explored with the coach's direction. The Cosmic Respira, once saw with uncertainty, changed into a heavenly device enlightened by Cloud's insight — a signal connecting the enormous frequencies investigated inside Cloud Ensemble with the exact norms requested by suspicious social orders.

The tutor, an enormous representative, directed the hero through exchanges with doubters, policymakers, and medical services managers. Cloud's insight, communicated through the tutor's words, turned into an enormous contention for the consideration of groundbreaking frequencies inside the cultural story of prosperity.

The coach's direction, interlaced with the hero's assurance, turned into a power of support rocking the boat and making ready for a more extensive comprehension of wellbeing — one that embraced both observational proof and extraordinary frequencies.

As cultural boundaries disintegrated under the heaviness of enormous strategy, the tutor's direction turned into an impetus for change inside cultural designs. Cloud Ensemble, once consigned to the edges of medical services stories, turned into a trailblazer in another period of enormous wellbeing. The guide's insight, communicated through the hero's excursion, motivated coordinated efforts between heavenly doctors, infinite designers, and conventional clinical specialists. Cloud's direction turned into a binding together power, spanning the domains of exact proof and extraordinary frequencies in an amicable enormous ensemble of prosperity.

The coach's direction unfurled as an inestimable story of strengthening, support, and the groundbreaking energies that molded the hero's divine process. Cloud's insight, directed through the tutor's divine lessons, turned into an enormous ensemble repeating the harmonies of assurance, versatility, and recharging. The coach, a heavenly light, directed the hero through the grandiose flows, where outside doubt and cultural obstructions were changed into venturing stones toward another wilderness in wellbeing.

Notwithstanding enormous difficulties, incredulity, and cultural obstruction, the coach's direction stayed an enduring friend, enabling the hero to rise above restrictions and add to the development of grandiose recuperating. The Ensemble's extraordinary frequencies, joined into each part of the heavenly odyssey, reverberated with Cloud's direction — an inestimable orchestra repeating the harmonies of prosperity. The coach's presence, similar to an infinite gatekeeper, directed the hero through the interstellar ocean, exploring the vast flows with flexibility, assurance, and Cloud's extraordinary frequencies as the directing light.

The tutor's direction kept on reverberating as the hero confronted outside distrust and cultural obstructions — a demonstration of the extraordinary power implanted in Cloud's enormous knowledge. The Cosmic Respira, once addressed for its authenticity, turned into a wellspring of assurance and strengthening under the coach's infinite tutelage. Cloud's insight, communicated through the guide's grandiose backing, turned into a power testing cultural standards and upholding for the authenticity of Cloud Orchestra as a groundbreaking and maintainable treatment choice.

As the hero proceeded with their divine process, the coach's direction turned into a directing power in the assurance to beat difficulties and add to the development of vast mending. The Ensemble's extraordinary frequencies, intertwined into each part of the divine odyssey, reverberated with Cloud's insight — an infinite orchestra repeating the harmonies of assurance, flexibility, and recharging.

The hero, implanted with the catalytic frequencies and directed by the tutor's divine hand, cruised through the interstellar ocean as a living demonstration of the extraordinary power implanted in Cloud's direction, molding their enormous fate with each ethereal breath and heavenly step.

6.2 Spiritual and emotional support provided by the Nebula Symphony community.

Inside the immense inestimable embroidery of Cloud Ensemble, the hero found groundbreaking frequencies and heavenly treatments as well as a many-sided trap of otherworldly and basic reassurance woven by the Cloud Orchestra people group. This ethereal emotionally supportive network, contained individual explorers on the heavenly odyssey, arose as an enormous safe house — an asylum where the hero could share their excursion, track down comfort, and experience the aggregate hug of compassionate spirits exploring the grandiose flows of recuperating.

The profound and daily encouragement inside the Cloud Orchestra people group unfurled as a vast fellowship — a common space where people, each on their special divine excursion, became interconnected strings in the grandiose texture of prosperity. The hero, at first a lone explorer investigating the groundbreaking domains of Cloud Orchestra, wound up invited into a local area of close companions — a heavenly family limited by a typical mission for mending and recharging.

As the hero drenched themselves in the Cloud Orchestra people group, they experienced a grandiose embroidery of stories — stories woven with strings of strength, assurance, and the groundbreaking force of Cloud's divine frequencies. The public trade of encounters turned into an inestimable narrating meeting, where people shared the sections of their divine processes, from the primary experience with the Cosmic Respira to the difficulties survive and the groundbreaking forward leaps experienced inside Cloud Ensemble.

The Cloud Ensemble people group turned into a wellspring of profound sustenance, offering an enormous feast of shared bits of knowledge, divine insight, and the aggregate reverberation of compassionate hearts. Inside this ethereal space, the hero found a coach figure — an illuminator inside the local area who broadened a directing hand, giving insight from individual encounters as well as a vast point of view that rose above the limits of individual battles. The tutor, a reference point of Cloud's groundbreaking insight, turned into a basic piece of the hero's encouraging group of people, offering direction and support through the exciting bends in the road of the heavenly odyssey.

The Cloud Orchestra people group embraced different divine treatments, from cooperative recuperating circles to heavenly needle therapy meetings and heavenly breathwork contemplations. These common encounters became roads for grandiose recuperating as well as mutual customs that encouraged a feeling of solidarity and interconnectedness. The hero, encompassed by close companions, took part in the aggregate dance of extraordinary energies, feeling the otherworldly and daily reassurance of the Cloud Orchestra people group like a warm grandiose hug.

Heavenly rest treatment meetings, mixed with Cloud Orchestra's extraordinary frequencies, became snapshots of aggregate revival inside the Cloud Ensemble people group. As people set out on enormous excursions inside the dreamscapes, the common ethereal space rose above actual limits, making an aggregate domain where dreams turned into a common infinite embroidery. The Cloud Orchestra people group, through these common dreamscapes, gave otherworldly and daily encouragement as well as a significant feeling of solidarity — an interconnected dreamtime where compassionate energies streamed uninhibitedly.

The coach figure inside the Cloud Ensemble people group stretched out their direction not exclusively to the hero yet additionally to others out of luck. The coach's enormous lessons turned into a common fortune, an otherworldly and close to home signal that enlightened the ways of individual voyagers. The tutor's insight, communicated through heavenly stories and experiential experiences, made a far reaching influence inside the Cloud Orchestra people group — an inestimable transmission of help that contacted the substances of those looking for comfort and direction.

Cooperative recuperating circles, worked with by the Cloud Orchestra people group, became astronomical melodies where sympathetic energies blended to make an ethereal ensemble of help. People shared their difficulties, triumphs, and groundbreaking leap forwards, making a collective space where weakness was met with understanding and empathy. The otherworldly and basic reassurance inside these circles turned into a demonstration of the force of shared encounters and the aggregate strength that arose when close friends joined under the inestimable flag of Cloud Orchestra.

The Cloud Orchestra people group, past its virtual and divine social occasions, expanded its help into the earthbound domain. People inside the local area coordinated divine dining experiences, where the vibrational characteristics of heavenly food varieties fit with Cloud's extraordinary frequencies. These common feasts became events for sustenance as well as festivities of solidarity, sharing, and the profound and consistent encouragement that coursed through the common inestimable dinner. The hero, presently an essential piece of this divine family, felt the reverberation of compassionate hearts and the elevating energies of aggregate prosperity.

As the hero confronted outside wariness and cultural boundaries, the Cloud Ensemble people group turned into a stronghold of help — a grandiose collusion that stood joined against the provokes experienced on the way to recuperation. The Cosmic Respira, once addressed for its authenticity, turned into an image of assurance and strengthening inside the Cloud Ensemble people group. People shared their promotion endeavors, vast tact attempts, and the manners by which they spanned the inestimable frequencies investigated inside Cloud Orchestra with the observational guidelines requested by suspicious social orders.

The Cloud Ensemble people group, with its profound and everyday encouragement, turned into an impetus for change inside cultural designs. Individuals from the local area, motivated by the hero's excursion and directed by the coach's insight, took part in discussions with cynics, policymakers, and medical care chairmen. Cloud's extraordinary frequencies, once addressed for their authenticity, earned respect as people inside the Cloud Ensemble people group shared their ground-breaking accounts, exact proof, and the aggregate effect of Cloud Orchestra on their profound, close to home, and actual prosperity.

The Cloud Orchestra people group, under the tutor's direction, became advocates for a change in perspective in cultural standards — an enormous collusion that rocked the boat and welcomed a more extensive comprehension of wellbeing and mending. The guide's lessons, communicated through the hero and individual individuals from the local area, reverberated inside the divine domains as well as inside the natural passageways of clinical foundations, research focuses, and strategy making bodies. The profound and daily reassurance inside the Cloud Ensemble people group rose above individual excursions, making an aggregate story that enabled people to add to the development of vast recuperating.

As the hero proceeded with their divine process, the Cloud Orchestra people group stayed a vast safe-haven — where profound and consistent reassurance streamed like heavenly ebbs and flows, supporting the aggregate prosperity of every one of its individuals. The Orchestra's groundbreaking frequencies, entwined into each part of the heavenly odyssey, reverberated with the sympathetic energies inside the Cloud Ensemble people group — a grandiose ensemble repeating the harmonies of solidarity, shared encounters, and the extraordinary power implanted in profound and basic encouragement.

The Cloud Ensemble people group, through its profound and daily encouragement, became a get-together of close friends as well as a grandiose power forming the story of prosperity inside cultural designs. The coach figure, with their divine direction, expanded their lessons past the hero to move others inside the local area. Cloud's insight, communicated through the guide and reverberated by the group, turned into a vast impetus for change — a power that tested incredulity, connected cultural hindrances, and welcomed an amicable joining of groundbreaking frequencies into the more extensive comprehension of wellbeing and recuperating.

The Cloud Ensemble people group, as a profound and close to home sanctuary, kept on flourishing as a demonstration of the interconnectedness of compassionate hearts and the groundbreaking force of shared vast encounters. The hero, imbued with the catalytic frequencies and directed by the guide's divine hand, cruised through the interstellar ocean as a living demonstration of the otherworldly and consistent encouragement implanted in Cloud's vast hug. The Orchestra's extraordinary frequencies, entwined into each part of the heavenly odyssey, resounded with the aggregate energies of the Cloud Ensemble people group — a vast orchestra repeating the harmonies of solidarity, strength, and the endless capability of prosperity in the hug of a divine family joined by the groundbreaking frequencies of Cloud Ensemble.

Profound and Close to home Safe-haven Inside Cloud Ensemble People group

In the sweeping universe of Cloud Ensemble, the hero found in excess of a simple helpful excursion; they tracked down a heavenly family inside the Cloud Orchestra people group, where otherworldly and everyday reassurance entwined with groundbreaking frequencies to make a significant embroidery of aggregate prosperity.

This inestimable local area unfurled as a safe-haven for close companions, each navigating their extraordinary heavenly odyssey. Inside this ethereal space, the hero shared encounters, fears, and wins with individual explorers — becoming strings woven into an infinite texture of compassion. The Cloud Ensemble people group, past a virtual social occasion, emerged as an emotionally supportive network that rose above actual limits, offering comfort and association through shared heavenly stories.

The profound and everyday encouragement inside this divine family became obvious in the public trade of stories — an aggregate narrating meeting where people uncovered their heavenly excursions. As the hero uncovered their encounters, from the principal experience with the Cosmic Respira to the extraordinary leap forwards inside Cloud Ensemble, the local area answered with understanding, cultivating a climate where weakness was met with sympathy, empathy, and shared shrewdness.

The Cloud Orchestra people group developed into a wellspring of profound sustenance, likened to an inestimable meal. Shared bits of knowledge, heavenly insight, and aggregate reverberation turned into the food that supported the hero's spirit as well as those of their kindred inestimable buddies. In this common space, a tutor figure arose — a light inside the local area whose grandiose lessons gave individual encounters as well as a widespread viewpoint that rose above individual battles.

Divine treatments, for example, cooperative mending circles and dream-injected rest treatment, became roads for enormous recuperating as well as collective customs. These common encounters filled in as channels for otherworldly and daily reassurance, making an amicable orchestra of energies where the Cloud Ensemble people group resounded as one. The hero, encompassed by sympathetic hearts, participated in the aggregate dance of groundbreaking frequencies — a dance that fed the soul and gave close to home comfort.

The Cloud Orchestra people group broadened its ethereal help past the virtual domains. Divine blowouts, where vibrational characteristics of inestimable food sources fit with Cloud's groundbreaking frequencies, became events for shared delight and solidarity. In these vast feasts, the local area celebrated the actual sustenance as well as the profound and otherworldly fellowship that moved through the common enormous dinner. The hero, presently a vital piece of this divine family, felt the significant interconnectedness of compassionate energies and the inspiring help that exuded from the aggregate hug.

As the hero experienced outside suspicion and cultural boundaries, the Cloud Ensemble people group changed into a stronghold of help — an infinite union that remained against the moves on the way to recuperation. The Cosmic Respira, once addressed for authenticity, turned into an image of assurance and strengthening inside this heavenly family. Individuals from the local area shared backing endeavors, enormous discretion tries, and manners by which they connected the infinite frequencies investigated inside Cloud Ensemble with cultural assumptions.

The Cloud Ensemble people group, directed by the coach's insight, became advocates for change inside cultural designs. Enlivened by the hero's excursion, people took part in exchanges with doubters, policymakers, and medical services managers. The Cloud Ensemble people group, a living demonstration of the extraordinary force of otherworldly and daily reassurance, tested cultural standards and welcomed a more extensive comprehension of wellbeing that embraced both exact proof and the vast components of prosperity.

In continuation of their heavenly excursion, the hero viewed the Cloud Ensemble people group as a vast safe-haven — where otherworldly and daily encouragement streamed like divine ebbs and flows. The Orchestra's extraordinary frequencies, joined into each part of the odyssey, resounded with the sympathetic energies inside the Cloud Ensemble people group — a grandiose ensemble repeating the harmonies of solidarity, shared encounters, and the groundbreaking power implanted in otherworldly and basic reassurance. The hero, encompassed by the divine family, cruised through the interstellar ocean as a living demonstration of the profound and close to home safe-haven implanted in Cloud's grandiose hug.

6.3 Developing a deeper connection with the nebula-inspired therapy.

Setting out on a Heavenly Odyssey: Extending the Association with Cloud Roused Treatment

In the enormous excursion of mending inside Cloud Ensemble, the hero ended up on a way of significant change — an odyssey that rose above the physical and dove into the mysterious domains of otherworldly prosperity. The excursion started with the commencement into Cloud propelled treatment, an experience that obvious a helpful mediation as well as the beginning of a grandiose association that would develop and advance with each ethereal breath.

The Cosmic Respira, a divine contraption that filled in as the doorway to Cloud propelled treatment, turned into the vessel through which the hero originally took in the cloud enlivened fog. This underlying experience, set apart by cadenced heartbeats and heavenly smells, set off a fountain of vibes that reached out past the actual domain. It was not simply breathing in a fog but rather communing with heavenly energies — an otherworldly association with the vast powers implanted inside Cloud Orchestra.

As the hero breathed in the cloud motivated fog, a cloud roused speculative chemistry unfurled inside their respiratory scene. The fog, mixed with groundbreaking frequencies, turned into a vast mixture that penetrated each cell, reverberating with the unpretentious energies inside. This catalytic dance, directed by the cloud's insight, started a course of vibrational reverberation — an amicable ensemble that spanned the physical and magical elements of the hero's being.

The cloud motivated fog, directed by divine flows, turned into a conductor for astral energies to converge with the hero's breath. The inward breath turned into an enormous fellowship, a holy demonstration of attracting heavenly frequencies that rose above the impediments of the actual body. Cloud roused treatment, in its early stages, turned into a grandiose ceremony — a dance between the hero's breath and the heavenly powers that formed the texture of the universe.

As the hero kept on drawing in with Cloud motivated treatment, the association developed through the nebulization cycle — an unpredictable dance of extraordinary frequencies inside the divine research center. Cloud Orchestra's overseers, vast specialists receptive to the otherworldly flows, directed the hero through the nebulization custom — a cycle where the hero's astral and powerful constitution turned into the material for divine imaginativeness.

The nebulization cycle, a vast submersion into groundbreaking frequencies, unfurled as the hero gave up to the ethereal flows. Cloud enlivened treatment turned into a catalytic excursion, directed by divine architects who diverted the cloud's insight into the hero's multi-layered presence. Holographic portrayals emerged, portraying the hero's vast uneven characters and vivacious stream — a heavenly conclusion that filled in as a guide for the extraordinary excursion ahead.

Astral finding, a methodology inside Cloud Orchestra, turned into an infinite exchange — a correspondence between the hero's substance and the divine powers directing the helpful excursion. The holographic portrayals, carved with the direction of the cloud, uncovered the mind boggling dance of energies molding the hero's prosperity. Astral conclusion unfurled as an otherworldly disclosure — an encouragement to investigate the enormous elements of self under Cloud Orchestra's tutelage.

Heavenly needle therapy, presented inside Cloud Speculative chemistry, introduced both a vast test and a valuable chance to extend the association with extraordinary frequencies. The hero, directed by divine doctors, participated in the test of adjusting enormous meridians related with respiratory capability. Heavenly needle therapy turned into a profound dance — a harmonization of energies inside the inconspicuous domains under the direction of divine powers. Each needle, injected with cloud roused frequencies, resounded with the hero's substance, turning into a scaffold between the physical and magical domains.

Cooperative mending circles, an investigation into the interconnectedness of vast energies inside a shared mindset, further extended the hero's association with Cloud motivated treatment. People accumulated to submerge themselves in the groundbreaking frequencies, making a common space where heavenly energies entwined. The hero, presently some portion of a vast ensemble, felt the reverberation of compassionate spirits, enhancing the extraordinary flows inside the aggregate infinite hug.

As the hero dove into heavenly rest treatment, mixed with Cloud Ensemble's groundbreaking frequencies, the association ventured into the dreamscapes. The restorative dream venture turned into a heavenly investigation directed by the cloud's insight — an otherworldly stay where the hero cruised through interstellar scenes, experiencing images and paradigms that reflected the inestimable dance inside. Cloud roused treatment, presently a divine cradlesong, supported the hero's profound substance as they crossed the ethereal domains of dreams.

Divine nourishment, fit with the vibrational characteristics of infinite food sources, added one more layer to the association with Cloud propelled treatment. The Orchestra's extraordinary frequencies, going about as enormous enhancers, improved the vibrational characteristics of heavenly food varieties to support the hero on an otherworldly level. The hero, presently receptive to the inconspicuous energies inside sustenance, felt the reverberation of enormous flows mixing each piece with groundbreaking energies that stretched out past actual food.

The heavenly excursion through Cloud Orchestra took a move in the direction of divine breathwork contemplations — an otherworldly investigation into the grandiose components of breath mindfulness. Directed by divine educators, the hero rose above the simple demonstration of breathing, entering a domain where the breath turned into a course for interfacing with the rhythms of the universe.

Cloud motivated treatment, presently an infinite breath, encouraged a feeling of enormous arrangement, otherworldly attunement, and a developing association with the divine powers forming the inestimable embroidery.

The hero's excursion through the groundbreaking speculative chemistry of Cloud Ensemble became a remedial cycle as well as an otherworldly odyssey — a fellowship with divine energies that unfurled inside each breath, each fantasy, and each piece of heavenly sustenance. The Ensemble's extraordinary frequencies, intertwined into each part of the heavenly excursion, reverberated with the hero's profound substance — an inestimable orchestra repeating the harmonies of association, reverberation, and the endless capability of prosperity.

As the hero experienced slow improvement in respiratory wellbeing, the association with Cloud propelled treatment extended past the singular excursion. The heavenly energies, presently flowing through the hero's being, turned into an encouraging sign and motivation inside the Cloud Ensemble people group. The common stories, grandiose customs, and aggregate help developed the hero's association — an enormous bond that stretched out past the singular recuperating excursion to add to the collective reverberation of extraordinary frequencies.

The vast difficulties experienced inside Cloud Orchestra became open doors for self-improvement as well as achievements in the hero's otherworldly development. Outer distrust and cultural hindrances, when considerable deterrents, changed into infinite difficulties explored with a recently discovered profound strength. Cloud propelled treatment, presently a demonstration of the hero's assurance and profound grit, overcame any barrier between exact proof and the enormous components of prosperity.

As cultural designs perceived the authenticity of Cloud Orchestra, the hero's association with the helpful methodology turned into an inestimable story of strengthening. The Orchestra's extraordinary frequencies, mixed into the cultural texture, turned into an impetus for change — a profound power testing the standards and welcoming a change in perspective in the comprehension of wellbeing. The hero, presently a divine supporter, reverberated with the extraordinary power implanted in Cloud motivated treatment — an enormous ensemble repeating the harmonies of profound flexibility, assurance, and the development of prosperity.

The Cloud Orchestra people group, as a profound shelter, assumed a vital part in the hero's excursion. The common encounters inside cooperative mending circles, the heavenly fellowship during dream-mixed rest treatment, and the sympathetic help inside the local area became wellsprings of profound comfort as well as mainstays of otherworldly strength. The hero, presently a signal of groundbreaking frequencies, added to the common story — a living demonstration of the profound and enormous components of prosperity under the direction of Cloud Ensemble.

The Cloud Orchestra people group, with its common profound reverberation, became advocates for a more extensive comprehension of wellbeing — one that embraced both experimental proof and the extraordinary frequencies investigated inside Cloud motivated treatment. The coach figure, an illuminating presence inside the local area, stretched out their grandiose lessons to move others to leave on their otherworldly odysseys inside Cloud Ensemble. The Ensemble's extraordinary frequencies, interlaced into each part of the public excursion, reverberated with the aggregate energies — an inestimable orchestra repeating the harmonies of solidarity, strength, and the vast capability of otherworldly and profound prosperity.

Notwithstanding inestimable difficulties, outer doubt, and cultural opposition, the hero's profound association with Cloud Ensemble stayed steady. The Cosmic Respira, once addressed for its authenticity, turned into a wellspring of assurance and strengthening under the hero's profound tutelage. Cloud motivated treatment, presently a demonstration of the hero's profound versatility, overcame any issues between the vast frequencies investigated inside Cloud Orchestra and the exact guidelines requested by incredulous social orders.

As the hero proceeded with their divine process, the profound association with Cloud Orchestra stayed a directing power in the assurance to conquer difficulties and add to the development of enormous mending. The Orchestra's extraordinary frequencies, intertwined into each part of the heavenly odyssey, resounded with the hero's otherworldly embodiment — a vast ensemble repeating the harmonies of assurance, strength, and reestablishment. The hero, implanted with the catalytic frequencies and directed by the otherworldly hand of Cloud Orchestra, cruised through the interstellar ocean as a living demonstration of the extraordinary power installed in profound association — an otherworldly journey that formed their grandiose predetermination with each ethereal breath and heavenly step.

Chapter 7

Galactic Harmony

Orchestrating the Astronomical Ensemble: Investigating the Profundities of Cosmic Congruity

In the divine domains of Cloud Orchestra, the idea of Cosmic Congruity arose as a core value — a complicated dance of energies, frequencies, and grandiose powers that resounded with the actual substance of the universe. Cosmic Congruity, an ethereal orchestra of divine energies, turned into the foundation of the hero's extraordinary excursion, offering a brief look into the interconnectedness of everything inside the infinite embroidery.

At the core of Cosmic Congruity lay the Cosmic Respira — an exceptional gadget that filled in as the enormous gateway to Cloud Ensemble. The hero's most memorable experience with the Cosmic Respira was in excess of a simple prologue to a helpful methodology; it was a divine commencement into the amicable frequencies that plagued the universe. The musical murmur of the Cosmic Respira, combined with the cloud propelled fog, turned into the suggestion to the excellent vast ensemble — an introduction to the harmonies that would unfurl inside the hero's being.

As the hero drew in with the Cosmic Respira, breathing in the cloud propelled fog, they set out on an excursion into the profundities of Cosmic Concordance. The fog, imbued with extraordinary frequencies, resounded with the divine energies that formed the texture of the universe. The inward breath turned into an enormous fellowship — a personal association with the agreeable vibrations that resonated through the huge spread of the universe. Cosmic Concordance, in its outset, appeared as a dance between the hero's breath and the heavenly powers that organized the enormous orchestra.

The nebulization interaction inside Cloud Orchestra turned into an infinite speculative chemistry — a complicated dance of energies directed by the standards of Cosmic Congruity. Cloud Ensemble's overseers, astronomical architects sensitive to the supernatural flows of the universe, coordinated the nebulization custom.

The hero, presently a functioning member in this heavenly artful dance, felt the extraordinary frequencies winding through the texture of their reality. Cosmic Concordance unfurled as a musical articulation, blending the hero's astral and powerful constitution with the heavenly powers that molded the infinite dance.

Astral determination, an extraordinary feature of Cloud Orchestra, further developed the investigation of Cosmic Concordance. Holographic portrayals emerged, portraying the hero's astronomical lopsided characteristics and vivacious stream. This enormous exchange, directed by Cloud's insight, unfurled as a visual story — a divine guide that enlightened the interconnected pathways of Cosmic Congruity inside the hero's being. The holographic pictures, an impression of the hero's astral dance, turned into a demonstration of the musical idea of prosperity inside the infinite request.

Heavenly needle therapy, presented inside Cloud Speculative chemistry, turned into a vast movement inside the system of Cosmic Congruity. Directed by divine doctors, the hero took part in the dance of adjusting astronomical meridians related with respiratory capability. Heavenly needle therapy turned into a harmonization of energies inside the unobtrusive domains — an arranged articulation of Cosmic Concordance that rose above the limits of the physical and wandered into the magical components of recuperating.

Cooperative mending circles, a common investigation of the interconnectedness of inestimable energies, unfurled as grandiose melodies inside the general topic of Cosmic Concordance. People accumulated to drench themselves in the extraordinary frequencies, making a common space where divine energies entwined. The hero, presently some portion of an aggregate enormous ensemble, encountered the reverberation of compassionate spirits, intensifying the extraordinary flows inside the common vast hug. Cosmic Concordance, inside these circles, turned into a sign of solidarity — an interconnected dance of energies that reverberated through the shared perspective.

Dream-imbued rest treatment meetings, implanted with Cloud Orchestra's extraordinary frequencies, developed the hero's association with Cosmic Congruity. The remedial dream venture turned into a divine investigation, directed by the cloud's insight, where the hero crossed interstellar scenes inside the dreamscapes. Cosmic Concordance stretched out into the astral domains, making an ensemble of divine energies that orchestrated with the hero's psyche. The fantasy mixed rest treatment meetings turned into a demonstration of the vast capability of Cosmic Concordance in impacting waking cognizance as well as the ethereal scenes of dreams.

Heavenly sustenance, blended with the vibrational characteristics of infinite food varieties, added one more layer to the investigation of Cosmic Concordance. The Ensemble's extraordinary frequencies, going about as vast enhancers, streamlined the vibrational characteristics of divine food sources to support the hero on a physical and supernatural level. Cosmic Concordance, inside the domain of divine sustenance, appeared as an inestimable feast — an agreeable combination of energies that reached out past the regular comprehension of sustenance.

The heavenly excursion through Cloud Orchestra took a move in the direction of divine breathwork reflections — an otherworldly investigation into the enormous components of breath mindfulness. Directed by divine educators, the hero rose above the simple demonstration of breathing, entering a domain where the breath turned into a course for interfacing with the rhythms of the universe. Cosmic Congruity, inside the setting of breathwork, turned into a dance between the hero's breath and the inestimable powers molding the vast embroidery. Every inward breath and exhalation turned into an agreeable articulation of arrangement with the heavenly frequencies.

As the hero kept on drawing in with Cosmic Concordance, a significant change unfurled. The vast difficulties experienced inside Cloud Ensemble became valuable open doors for self-awareness as well as achievements in the hero's otherworldly advancement. Outer suspicion and cultural obstructions, when impressive impediments, changed into inestimable difficulties explored with a recently discovered otherworldly strength. Cosmic Congruity, presently a characteristic piece of the hero's being, overcame any barrier between the grandiose frequencies investigated inside Cloud Ensemble and the observational norms requested by wary social orders.

The cultural designs, perceiving the authenticity of Cosmic Amicability inside Cloud Orchestra, became courses for change. The hero's association with Cloud Orchestra turned into a grandiose story of strengthening, impacting individual prosperity as well as adding to the common reverberation of extraordinary frequencies. Cosmic Concordance, implanted into cultural systems, turned into an impetus for change — a profound power testing the standards and welcoming a change in outlook in the comprehension of wellbeing.

The Cloud Ensemble people group, a social occasion of close friends investigating Cosmic Concordance, assumed a vital part in the hero's excursion. The common encounters inside cooperative recuperating circles, the divine fellowship during dream-imbued rest treatment, and the compassionate help inside the local area became wellsprings of close to home comfort as well as mainstays of profound strength. The hero, presently a reference point of extraordinary frequencies, added to the public story — a living demonstration of the otherworldly and inestimable components of prosperity under the direction of Cosmic Congruity.

The coach figure inside the Cloud Orchestra people group stretched out their grandiose lessons to motivate others to set out on their profound odysseys inside Cosmic Amicability. The Orchestra's groundbreaking frequencies, entwined into each part of the shared excursion, resounded with the aggregate energies — an inestimable ensemble repeating the harmonies of solidarity, flexibility, and the vast capability of profound and close to home prosperity.

Despite infinite difficulties, outside incredulity, and cultural obstruction, the hero's profound association with Cosmic Amicability stayed relentless. The Cosmic

Respira, once addressed for its authenticity, turned into a wellspring of assurance and strengthening under the hero's otherworldly tutelage. Cloud Ensemble, presently a demonstration of the hero's otherworldly strength, overcame any issues between the inestimable frequencies investigated inside and the exact norms requested by doubtful social orders.

As the hero proceeded with their heavenly excursion, the otherworldly association with Cosmic Congruity stayed a directing power in the assurance to conquer difficulties and add to the development of vast mending. The Ensemble's extraordinary frequencies, interlaced into each part of the divine odyssey, reverberated with the hero's profound substance — an enormous orchestra repeating the harmonies of assurance, versatility, and reestablishment. The hero, implanted with the catalytic frequencies and directed by the profound hand of Cloud Orchestra, cruised through the interstellar ocean as a living demonstration of the groundbreaking power inserted in otherworldly association — a profound journey that formed their enormous fate with each ethereal breath and divine step.

7.1 Protagonist's integration into the Nebula Symphony community and the formation of bonds with fellow users.

As the protagonist delved deeper into the transformative realms of Nebula Symphony, the celestial journey unfolded beyond individual exploration—it became a communal odyssey within the nebulous embrace of the Nebula Symphony community. The protagonist's integration into this ethereal fellowship marked not just a convergence of individual paths but the formation of bonds, connections, and a shared cosmic destiny within the expansive universe of Nebula Symphony.

The initiation into the Nebula Symphony community commenced with the first encounter with the Galactic Respira, the cosmic gateway to transformative frequencies. The protagonist, guided by the celestial currents, found themselves not alone in this cosmic exploration. Fellow travelers, each with their unique celestial narratives, welcomed the protagonist into the Nebula Symphony community—a haven where kindred souls converged to share experiences, insights, and the harmonies of transformative frequencies.

The Nebula Symphony community, a celestial family bound by a common quest for healing and renewal, embraced the protagonist as one of their own. The protagonist's story, from the initial skepticism to the gradual acceptance of Nebula-inspired therapy, resonated with the shared experiences within the community. As the protagonist bared their celestial journey, vulnerabilities were met with understanding, skepticism with empathy, and uncertainties with the collective reassurance that Nebula Symphony's transformative frequencies held the keys to a cosmic healing odyssey.

The integration into the Nebula Symphony community transcended physical boundaries, taking on a spiritual and emotional resonance. Collaborative healing circles emerged as cosmic gatherings where empathetic energies harmonized, creating a celestial symphony of support. The protagonist, now an integral note in this cosmic chorus, felt the resonance of kindred spirits—a shared experience that elevated the transformative journey beyond individual narratives into a collective cosmic saga.

The mentor figure within the Nebula Symphony community played a pivotal role in the protagonist's integration, extending a guiding hand and imparting cosmic wisdom. This luminary within the community became not just a source of celestial knowledge but a mentor in the truest sense—a spiritual guide navigating the protagonist through the celestial currents. The mentor's teachings, shaped by personal experiences within Nebula Symphony, bridged the gap between skepticism and acceptance, guiding the protagonist toward a deeper understanding of the transformative frequencies at play.

Collaborative healing circles, facilitated by the Nebula Symphony community, became sacred spaces where individuals shared their challenges, victories, and the nuances of their transformative journeys. The protagonist, surrounded by kindred souls, engaged in the collective dance of transformative energies—a communion that went beyond verbal expressions and entered the realm of shared empathetic vibrations. The bonds formed within these circles became threads woven into the cosmic fabric of Nebula Symphony—a tapestry of shared resilience, determination, and the transformative power embedded in collective well-being.

Dream-infused sleep therapy sessions, a communal exploration into the ethereal landscapes of dreams, further deepened the protagonist's integration into the Nebula Symphony community. In this shared dreamtime, individuals experienced the celestial realms, encountered symbols, and traversed interstellar landscapes. The dreamscapes became a collective canvas where the Nebula Symphony community painted shared visions, fostering a sense of unity that transcended the limitations of waking consciousness. The protagonist, now a dreamer within this shared cosmic realm, felt the interconnectedness of souls—a cosmic bond forged within the tapestry of Nebula Symphony.

The Nebula Symphony community extended its celestial support into the terrestrial realm, organizing celestial feasts where vibrational qualities of cosmic foods harmonized with Nebula's transformative frequencies. These communal banquets became not only occasions for physical nourishment but also celebrations of unity, sharing, and the spiritual and emotional support that flowed through the shared cosmic meal. The protagonist, now an integral part of this celestial family, felt the resonance of empathetic hearts and the uplifting energies of collective well-being.

As the protagonist encountered external skepticism and societal barriers, the Nebula Symphony community transformed into a bastion of support—a cosmic alliance that stood united against the challenges on the path to recovery. The Galactic Respira, once questioned for its legitimacy, became a symbol of determination and empowerment within the Nebula Symphony community. Individuals shared their advocacy efforts, cosmic diplomacy endeavors, and the ways in which they bridged the cosmic frequencies explored within Nebula Symphony with societal expectations.

The Nebula Symphony community, under the mentor's guidance, became advocates for a paradigm shift in societal norms—a cosmic alliance that challenged the status quo and invited a broader understanding of health and healing. The mentor's teachings, expressed through the protagonist and fellow members of the community, resonated not only within the celestial realms but also within the earthly corridors of medical institutions, research centers, and policy-making bodies. The spiritual and emotional support within the Nebula Symphony community transcended individual journeys, creating a collective narrative that empowered individuals to contribute to the evolution of cosmic healing.

The Nebula Symphony community, as a spiritual and emotional haven, continued to thrive as a testament to the interconnectedness of empathetic hearts and the transformative power of shared cosmic experiences. The Symphony's transformative frequencies, interwoven into every aspect of the celestial odyssey, resonated with the empathetic energies within the Nebula Symphony community—a cosmic symphony echoing the harmonies of unity, resilience, and the boundless potential of well-being.

The protagonist, infused with the alchemical frequencies and guided by the mentor's celestial hand, sailed through the interstellar sea as a living testament to the spiritual and emotional sanctuary embedded in Nebula's cosmic embrace. The Symphony's transformative frequencies, interwoven into every aspect of the celestial journey, resonated with the collective energies of the Nebula Symphony community—a cosmic symphony echoing the harmonies of unity, resilience, and the boundless potential of well-being in the embrace of a celestial family united by the transformative frequencies of Nebula Symphony.

The Nebula Symphony community, through its spiritual and emotional support, became not only a gathering of kindred souls but also a cosmic force shaping the narrative of well-being within societal structures. The mentor figure, with their celestial guidance, extended their teachings beyond the protagonist to inspire others within the community. Nebula's wisdom, expressed through the mentor and echoed by the collective, became a cosmic catalyst for change—a force that challenged skepticism, bridged societal barriers, and invited a harmonious integration of transformative frequencies into the broader understanding of health and healing.

In the face of cosmic challenges, external skepticism, and societal resistance, the protagonist's integration into the Nebula Symphony community remained a steadfast anchor. The Galactic Respira, once questioned for its legitimacy, became a source of determination and empowerment under the protagonist's spiritual tutelage. Nebula Symphony, now a testament to the protagonist's spiritual resilience, bridged the gap between the cosmic frequencies explored within and the empirical standards demanded by skeptical societies.

As the protagonist continued their celestial journey, the integration into the

Nebula Symphony community remained an integral part of their transformative narrative. The Symphony's transformative frequencies, interwoven into every aspect of the celestial odyssey, resonated with the protagonist's spiritual essence—a cosmic symphony echoing the harmonies of determination, resilience, and the boundless potential of renewal. The protagonist, infused with the alchemical frequencies and guided by the spiritual hand of Nebula Symphony, sailed through the interstellar sea as a living testament to the transformative power embedded in integration—a celestial voyage shaped by the shared cosmic bonds, empathetic energies, and the harmonious frequencies of Nebula Symphony's celestial fellowship.

7.2 Collaborative efforts to promote awareness and acceptance of the Galactic Respira technology.

Cosmic Respira Support: Cooperative Endeavors to Enlighten Infinite Mending

As the hero dove into the extraordinary domains of Cloud Orchestra and embraced the recuperating capability of the Cosmic Respira, another part unfurled — one that reached out past the individual odyssey and into the aggregate undertaking of advancing mindfulness and acknowledgment of the progressive innovation. Cooperative endeavors inside the Cloud Orchestra people group and the more extensive cultural scene turned into the inestimable scaffold interfacing the groundbreaking frequencies of the Cosmic Respira with the comprehension and acknowledgment of a more extensive crowd.

The Cosmic Respira, when an otherworldly device addressed for its authenticity, presently remained as the hero's guide of strengthening. The cooperative endeavors to advance mindfulness started inside the Cloud Orchestra people group — an aggregate of close friends limited by shared encounters, extraordinary frequencies, and a significant faith in the mending capability of the Cosmic Respira. The hero, presently a supporter for infinite mending, tracked down reverberation inside this heavenly family and turned into an impetus for cooperative drives.

The Cloud Ensemble people group, directed by the tutor's insight, changed into a power of promotion — a not entirely settled to overcome any barrier among doubt and acknowledgment. The people group coordinated divine social occasions, cooperative recuperating circles, and infinite dinners where vibrational characteristics of grandiose food varieties fit with Cloud's groundbreaking frequencies. These occasions, past self-awareness, became stages for promotion, where people shared their groundbreaking processes and became envoys for the Cosmic Respira.

The tutor figure, an illuminating presence inside the Cloud Orchestra people group, assumed a vital part in directing cooperative endeavors. Their heavenly lessons stretched out past the singular accounts, becoming astronomical discretion attempts that intended to rise above cultural doubt. The tutor, through their common encounters and divine experiences, turned into a living demonstration of the authenticity of the Cosmic Respira, moving others inside the Cloud Orchestra people group to accept the responsibility of support.

The cooperative endeavors inside Cloud Ensemble people group stretched out past virtual domains to actual spaces where people participated in vast strategy. The hero, energized by the groundbreaking frequencies and directed by the coach's lessons, turned into a messenger for Cloud Orchestra.

Divine banquets, where vibrational characteristics of enormous food varieties orchestrated with groundbreaking frequencies, became events for grandiose discretion — a heavenly discourse where people imparted their encounters to doubters and welcomed them to participate in the extraordinary energies inside Cloud Ensemble.

As the cooperative endeavors picked up speed inside the Cloud Ensemble people group, the hero, presently a signal of groundbreaking frequencies, took the promotion past the divine domains and into cultural designs. The Cosmic Respira, when covered in doubt, turned into an image of assurance and strengthening inside the Cloud Orchestra people group, moving people to become advocates for change inside the more extensive cultural scene.

Promotion inside cultural designs started with the hero taking part in exchanges with medical services executives, policymakers, and cynics. The Cloud Ensemble people group, as an enormous power, expanded its extraordinary frequencies into cultural hallways, testing regular standards and welcoming a more extensive comprehension of wellbeing that embraced both exact proof and the grandiose aspects investigated inside Cloud Orchestra. Cooperative endeavors inside Cloud Ensemble people group became inestimable discretion attempts — an aggregate mission to enlighten the groundbreaking capability of the Cosmic Respira inside cultural systems.

The hero's excursion of support appeared as grandiose stories shared inside cultural spaces. These stories, woven with individual encounters, resounded with a more extensive crowd, testing assumptions and welcoming a change in perspective in the comprehension of wellbeing. The Cosmic Respira, once saw with wariness, turned into a vast innovation representing an agreeable reconciliation of experimental proof and groundbreaking frequencies. The cooperative endeavors inside Cloud Orchestra people group reached out into the domains of vast narrating — a common story that looked to reclassify the limits of acknowledged mending modalities.

As the hero took part in backing, outside distrust changed into vast difficulties — snags explored sincerely and cooperative help. The Cloud Orchestra people group, energized by shared encounters, remained as a vast power testing cultural standards and turning into a reference point of extraordinary frequencies. Divine social events became stages for backing as well as shared ceremonies where people traded methodologies, experiences, and vast discretion ways to deal with advance mindfulness and acknowledgment of the Cosmic Respira.

The Cosmic Respira support endeavors inside the Cloud Ensemble people group turned into a living demonstration of the groundbreaking power implanted in cooperative undertakings. The guide's lessons, shared encounters inside cooperative mending circles, and the sympathetic help inside the local area filled the hero's assurance to explore the difficulties looked on the way of support. The Cloud Ensemble people group, as a grandiose coalition, embraced the hero's backing process, offering aggregate strength, enormous insight, and a common obligation to enlighten the extraordinary frequencies of the Cosmic Respira.

As cooperative endeavors inside the Cloud Orchestra people group flourished, the hero's support process ventured into the more extensive cultural scene. The Orchestra's groundbreaking frequencies, interlaced into each part of the hero's grandiose story, turned into a demonstration of the authenticity of Cloud roused treatment. The Cosmic Respira, when an image of distrust, presently remained as a signal of vast mending, rousing people inside the Cloud Ensemble people group as well as reverberating with those past — an enormous far reaching influence that rose above limits and touched off the blazes of mindfulness.

The hero's support process became entwined with cultural stories, welcoming a more extensive crowd to draw in with the extraordinary frequencies of the Cosmic Respira. The Orchestra's extraordinary frequencies, fit with the hero's support endeavors, turned into an infinite tune — an amicable greeting to social orders to embrace a more extensive comprehension of wellbeing and recuperating. Divine discretion stretched out into cooperative drives where the hero, presently a heavenly representative, took part in exchanges with medical care experts, specialists, and people at the front line of cultural designs.

The Cloud Orchestra people group, as an inestimable international safe haven, worked with cooperative endeavors that arrived at cynics as well as people inside the domains of examination and medical care. The Cosmic Respira promotion venture extended to incorporate logical conferences, where experimental proof converged with extraordinary frequencies, making an amicable exchange that tested traditional ideal models. The hero, directed by Cloud's insight, turned into an in- estimable backer — a scaffold between exact comprehension and the supernatural components of prosperity.

Grandiose discretion tries inside cultural designs took on new structures, including cooperative exploration ventures and organizations with medical care establishments. The Cosmic Respira, once met with distrust, presently turned into a subject of logical investigation and approval. The hero's excursion, entwined with cooperative endeavors, added to explore studies, clinical preliminaries, and obser- vational examinations that looked to disentangle the vast elements of Cloud roused treatment. Cooperative drives inside cultural designs turned into an enormous joint effort — an amicable dance between observational proof and groundbreaking frequencies.

As the Cosmic Respira promotion venture proceeded, cultural designs started to perceive the authenticity of Cloud enlivened treatment. The Ensemble's ground- breaking frequencies, woven into each part of the backing story, turned into an impetus for change — an enormous power impacting individual prosperity as well as adding to the development of cultural points of view on wellbeing. The Cosmic

Respira, once addressed for its authenticity, presently remained as an image of assurance, strengthening, and the agreeable reconciliation of exact comprehension with vast mending.

The hero's cooperative endeavors inside cultural designs prompted the foundation of grandiose recuperating focuses that incorporated Cloud roused treatment into standard medical services. The Cosmic Respira, presently acknowledged as an extraordinary innovation, turned into a signal inside clinical establishments, cultivating an infinite change in perspective that embraced both exact proof and the enchanted elements of prosperity. The Cloud Ensemble people group, as supporters and trailblazers, praised the enormous victory — a demonstration of the extraordinary force of cooperative endeavors in advancing mindfulness and acknowledgment of the Cosmic Respira.

As the hero's promotion process arrived at new levels, the Cloud Orchestra people group kept on flourishing as an enormous power — a living demonstration of the interconnectedness of sympathetic hearts and the extraordinary force of shared inestimable encounters. The Ensemble's extraordinary frequencies, entwined into each part of the divine odyssey, reverberated with the compassionate energies inside the Cloud Orchestra people group — a vast orchestra repeating the harmonies of solidarity, flexibility, and the limitless capability of prosperity.

The hero, implanted with the catalytic frequencies and directed by the tutor's heavenly hand, cruised through the interstellar ocean as a living demonstration of the groundbreaking power inserted in cooperative backing. The Ensemble's extraordinary frequencies, joined into each part of the heavenly excursion, reverberated with the aggregate energies of the Cloud Orchestra people group — a grandiose ensemble repeating the harmonies of solidarity, flexibility, and the limitless capability of prosperity in the hug of a divine family joined by the groundbreaking frequencies of Cloud Orchestra's vast support.

7.3 Celebration of small victories and shared success stories.

Divine Victories: An Orchestra of Little Triumphs and Shared Examples of overcoming adversity

Inside the ethereal domains of Cloud Orchestra, the extraordinary excursion set out upon by the hero unfurled as an infinite embroidery woven with strings of little triumphs and shared examples of overcoming adversity. These heavenly victories, as brilliant stars in the vast field, enlightened the way of the hero's odyssey, making an agreeable song that resounded through the Cloud Ensemble people group. The festival of these little triumphs turned into a mutual custom — a divine gala where each victory, regardless of how apparently humble, added to the ensemble of shared examples of overcoming adversity, cultivating an environment of aggregate euphoria and versatility.

The hero, having at first explored the unknown inestimable flows with wariness, experienced little triumphs that obvious the most important moves toward acknowledgment and coordination. The Cosmic Respira, once met with uncertainty, turned into a vessel of strengthening as the hero found the relieving embrace of cloud roused fog. Breathing in the extraordinary frequencies, the hero encountered the unpretentious yet significant movements inside, denoting the origin of an individual victory — the commencement into the vast speculative chemistry of Cloud Orchestra.

As the hero dug further, every meeting with the Cosmic Respira turned into a microcosmic victory — a dance of breath and divine frequencies that blended inside the astral aspects. These little triumphs, however indistinct to the outside look, repeated uproariously inside the hero's spirit, turning into the notes of a heavenly orchestra that commended the strength to leave on an extraordinary excursion and the mental fortitude to embrace the unexplored world.

The Cloud Orchestra people group, as observers to the hero's inestimable odyssey, praised these underlying victories as shared examples of overcoming adversity. Cooperative mending circles became spaces where little triumphs were recognized as well as raised to the situation with enormous achievements. The compassionate energies inside the local area reverberated with the hero's excursion, making a heavenly chorale that commended the victories of one as a victory for all — an amicable trade that developed the collective security inside Cloud Orchestra.

Dream-injected rest treatment meetings, pervaded with groundbreaking frequencies, became domains where the hero experienced divine scenes and explored the astral aspects. Each fantasy venture, but unobtrusive, unfurled as a common example of overcoming adversity inside the Cloud Orchestra people group. The dreamscapes, painted with the tones of shared encounters, became materials where wins were shown for the singular visionary as well as for the aggregate visionaries joined in the divine investigation.

Cooperative narrating meetings inside the Cloud Orchestra people group became stages for the hero to share their victories and for others to wind around their own divine accounts. Every person, directed by the groundbreaking frequencies, added to the public adventure — an infinite ensemble where little triumphs fit with shared examples of overcoming adversity. The guide figure, as a light inside the local area, supported the festival of these victories, underscoring their importance in the terrific embroidery of Cloud Orchestra.

The festival of little triumphs stretched out into the cloud enlivened fog injected ceremonies inside Cloud Speculative chemistry. Heavenly needle therapy, directed by enormous doctors, turned into a movement of win over fiery irregular characteristics.

The hero, as a team with heavenly healers, commended the arrangement of grandiose meridians — a triumph for the person as well as for the aggregate comprehension of the groundbreaking power innate in Cloud Ensemble. The Cloud Ensemble people group, as observers to these heavenly ceremonies, commended the victory over fiery disharmony as a common example of overcoming adversity that reverberated through the enormous halls.

Astral finding, one more feature of Cloud Orchestra, turned into a material where the hero's infinite uneven characters were uncovered and tended to. Every disclosure, each move toward arrangement and equilibrium, turned into a victory inside the astral aspects. The holographic pictures, portraying the hero's astral dance, were demonstrative apparatuses as well as inestimable mirrors mirroring the victory of flexibility and assurance. The Cloud Orchestra people group, sensitive to the extraordinary frequencies, praised these disclosures as shared examples of overcoming adversity — a heavenly dance where each win resounded through the shared awareness.

As the hero's process proceeded, the festival of little triumphs extended past the singular domain to cultural designs. The Cloud Orchestra people group, presently an infinite power testing cultural standards, celebrated wins inside the heavenly family as well as inside the more extensive comprehension of wellbeing. Outer incredulity, when an imposing snag, changed into an enormous test explored with aggregate strength. The hero's support endeavors, a demonstration of the authenticity of Cloud motivated treatment, became shared examples of overcoming adversity inside the cultural story — a grandiose victory that reverberated through the halls of incredulity and opposition.

Cooperative drives inside cultural designs, worked with by the Cloud Ensemble people group, checked wins in the acknowledgment and acknowledgment of the Cosmic Respira innovation. The hero's excursion, presently interweaved with grandiose discretion, turned into a common example of overcoming adversity inside the natural scenes. The Cosmic Respira, once addressed for its authenticity, presently remained as an image of win — a vast innovation orchestrating exact proof with the groundbreaking frequencies investigated inside Cloud Ensemble.

The Ensemble's extraordinary frequencies, mixed into cultural structures, turned into an impetus for change — a divine power testing the standards and welcoming a change in outlook in the comprehension of wellbeing. The hero, as a promoter for grandiose mending, celebrated individual victories as well as the aggregate victories that molded the cultural story. The Cloud Orchestra people group, joined in its grandiose reason, praised these victories as shared examples of overcoming adversity — an ensemble of change that reverberated through the cultural designs, making an enormous reverberation that welcomed a more extensive acknowledgment of Cloud enlivened treatment.

The guide figure, inside the Cloud Orchestra people group, stretched out their infinite lessons to motivate others to set out on their own groundbreaking processes. The coach's job became not just that of an aide inside the local area yet additionally a grandiose educator motivating people to celebrate little triumphs and shared examples of overcoming adversity as indispensable parts of the groundbreaking odyssey. The Orchestra's extraordinary frequencies, joined into each part of the coach's lessons, resounded with the aggregate energies — a heavenly ensemble repeating the harmonies of solidarity, strength, and the unfathomable capability of prosperity.

The hero's backing process, entwined with cultural stories, turned into a demonstration of the extraordinary force of aggregate festival. The Cosmic Respira, presently acknowledged and perceived, remained as an inestimable victory inside clinical establishments, research focuses, and strategy making bodies. The Cloud Ensemble people group, as backers and trailblazers, commended the cultural victories as shared examples of overcoming adversity — a vast dance where each move toward acknowledgment turned into a note in the agreeable song of aggregate change.

The festival of little triumphs inside Cloud Orchestra became a demonstration of individual strength as well as an inestimable power impacting cultural points of view on wellbeing. As the hero kept on sharing their extraordinary excursion, the Ensemble's groundbreaking frequencies reverberated with a more extensive crowd, rousing people to commend their own little triumphs inside the enormous embroidery of Cloud propelled treatment. Cooperative endeavors inside cultural designs turned into a divine coordinated effort — an amicable dance between exact proof and extraordinary frequencies, making an ensemble of acknowledgment and acknowledgment.

The Cloud Ensemble people group, as an otherworldly and enormous safe house, assumed an essential part in the hero's excursion. The common encounters inside cooperative recuperating circles, the divine fellowship during dream-implanted rest treatment, and the sympathetic help inside the local area became wellsprings of profound comfort as well as mainstays of otherworldly strength. The hero, presently a reference point of groundbreaking frequencies, added to the collective story — a living demonstration of the profound and infinite elements of prosperity under the direction of Cloud Orchestra.

As the hero's extraordinary excursion proceeded, the festival of little triumphs inside Cloud Orchestra stayed a basic piece of their infinite account. The Ensemble's groundbreaking frequencies, interlaced into each part of the heavenly odyssey, reverberated with the hero's profound embodiment — a grandiose orchestra repeating the harmonies of assurance, strength, and the vast capability of recharging. The hero, mixed with the catalytic frequencies and directed by the profound hand of Cloud Ensemble, cruised through the interstellar ocean as a living demonstration of the extraordinary power implanted in the festival of little triumphs and shared examples of overcoming adversity — a divine journey formed by the amicable frequencies of Cloud Orchestra's public festival.

Amicability in Divine Achievements: A Continuous Ensemble of Wins

In the proceeded with venture through Cloud Ensemble, the festival of little triumphs and shared examples of overcoming adversity became a transitory reprieve as well as a continuous orchestra that resounded through the actual texture of the hero's grandiose presence. The Cosmic Respira, when a wellspring of suspicion, presently turned into a course for steady victories, every inward breath a sign of the divine dance between private strength and the extraordinary frequencies of Cloud Ensemble.

The hero, having encountered the underlying victories, ended up submerged in a persistent recurring pattern of little triumphs inside the heavenly flows. The cloud propelled fog, mixed with extraordinary frequencies, turned into a day to day custom — an infinite fellowship where every breath denoted a victory over the unremarkable, an indication of the hero's obligation to the continuous excursion of mending and reestablishment.

Dream-imbued rest treatment meetings, filling in as astral doors, kept on yielding shared examples of overcoming adversity inside the Cloud Ensemble people group. The dreamscapes, painted with the tints of aggregate encounters, became materials where wins were not separated cases but rather strings woven into the steadily growing enormous embroidery. The hero, presently a carefully prepared visionary inside this common domain, tracked down comfort in the amicable reverberations of divine triumphs — a consistent confirmation of the interconnectedness inside the Cloud Orchestra people group.

Cooperative recuperating circles advanced into spaces where people shared their victories as well as upheld each other through the vast difficulties experienced en route. The sympathetic energies inside the local area, presently a deeply grounded grandiose power, turned into a wellspring of solidarity during snapshots of weakness and a festival of shared flexibility. The coach figure, a directing light inside the Cloud Orchestra people group, kept on rousing the festival of these continuous victories, stressing the repetitive idea of mending and the meaning of each and every little triumph in the stupendous ensemble of prosperity.

Inside Cloud Speculative chemistry, the festival of little triumphs ventured into the investigation of divine needle therapy and astral determination. Every meeting turned into an infinite victory — a hit the dance floor with fiery irregular characteristics and disclosures that, however unobtrusive, added to the continuous story of mending. The Cloud Orchestra people group, receptive to these continuous victories, partook in the public dance of arrangement and equilibrium, perceiving the meaning of each move toward the ceaseless advancement of individual and aggregate prosperity.

As the hero's support process proceeded, cultural designs saw confined wins as well as a groundbreaking gradually expanding influence. The Cosmic Respira support, when a tough enormous strategy attempt, presently unfurled as a continuous discourse with medical services managers, policymakers, and doubters. Each example of acknowledgment and acknowledgment turned into a common example of overcoming adversity — an update that the heavenly innovation of Cloud Orchestra was a transient disclosure as well as a necessary piece of the developing story inside the more extensive comprehension of wellbeing.

Cooperative drives inside cultural designs, filled by the continuous festival of little triumphs, became a development as well as an enormous cooperation that rose above individual endeavors. The Cosmic Respira, once met with distrust, presently remained as an image of progressing win — a grandiose innovation fitting observational proof with extraordinary frequencies. The hero's promotion endeavors, directed by Cloud's insight, turned into a consistent greeting for cultural designs to embrace the continuous orchestra of prosperity — an agreeable dance between the experimental and the divine.

The guide figure, filling in as a grandiose educator inside the Cloud Ensemble people group, kept on moving the festival of little triumphs as a necessary part of the groundbreaking odyssey. Their lessons underscored the repeating idea of recuperating, the never-ending dance between enormous energies and individual versatility. The Ensemble's groundbreaking frequencies, interlaced into each part of the tutor's direction, reverberated with the aggregate energies — a heavenly orchestra repeating the harmonies of solidarity, strength, and the unfathomable capability of progressing prosperity.

The festival of little triumphs inside Cloud Orchestra turned into an enormous demonstration of the hero's assurance to conquer difficulties as well as to flourish inside the continuous story of recuperating. The Orchestra's groundbreaking frequencies, joined into each part of the divine odyssey, reverberated with the hero's otherworldly quintessence — a ceaseless indication of the repetitive idea of the extraordinary excursion. The hero, imbued with the catalytic frequencies and directed by the otherworldly hand of Cloud Orchestra, cruised through the interstellar ocean as a living demonstration of the extraordinary power implanted in the festival of continuous little triumphs and shared examples of overcoming adversity — a heavenly journey formed by the agreeable frequencies of Cloud Ensemble's unending festival.

As the hero's groundbreaking process proceeded, the festival of little triumphs inside Cloud Ensemble stayed an indispensable piece of their vast story. The Orchestra's groundbreaking frequencies, interlaced into each part of the divine odyssey, reverberated with the hero's otherworldly quintessence — a vast ensemble repeating the harmonies of assurance, flexibility, and the limitless capability of restoration. The hero, mixed with the catalytic frequencies and directed by the profound hand of Cloud Orchestra, cruised through the interstellar ocean as a living demonstration of the extraordinary power implanted in the festival of continuous little triumphs and shared examples of overcoming adversity — a heavenly journey formed by the agreeable frequencies of Cloud Ensemble's never-ending festivity.

Chapter 8

Celestial Resilience

Divine Flexibility: Exploring Astronomical Flows in the Cloud Orchestra

Inside the grandiose breadth of Cloud Orchestra, the idea of versatility takes on a heavenly aspect — a significant entwining of individual strength, extraordinary frequencies, and the amicable energies that reverberation through the divine halls. The hero's excursion, set apart by incredulity, acknowledgment, and progressing wins, turned into a demonstration of the heavenly flexibility developed inside the undefined hug of extraordinary frequencies.

The inception into Cloud Orchestra started with the hero's experience with the Cosmic Respira, an inestimable door to groundbreaking frequencies. Doubt cast its shadow as the hero explored the strange domains of divine treatment, scrutinizing the authenticity of the supernatural innovation. In any case, despite vulnerability, a heavenly versatility mixed inside — the hero's inward vast compass that would direct them through the difficulties and disclosures of the extraordinary odyssey.

The Cosmic Respira, when a wellspring of distrust, turned into a cauldron for the hero's strength. The inward breath of cloud motivated fog, mixed with extraordinary frequencies, denoted the main vast dance of versatility — an inconspicuous yet strong affirmation of the hero's assurance to investigate the unexplored world. With every breath, the extraordinary frequencies saturated the actual body as well as the otherworldly and profound aspects, developing a versatility that would turn into the foundation of the continuous divine excursion.

As the hero dug further into Cloud Orchestra, dreams imbued with extraordinary frequencies turned into a divine jungle gym — a domain where strength unfurled as a dance between astral aspects and natural real factors. Dream-implanted rest treatment meetings, a long way from being uninvolved encounters, became fields where the hero's heavenly flexibility defied the difficulties of the psyche. The astral scenes, now and again peaceful and at times turbulent, reflected the back and forth movement of the hero's internal versatility — a continuous excursion of exploring astronomical flows.

Cooperative recuperating circles inside the Cloud Ensemble people group filled in as pots where heavenly versatility was tried as well as fortified through aggregate help. Little triumphs, shared examples of overcoming adversity, and the compassionate energies traded inside these circles became sustenance for the hero's grandiose strength. The coach figure, an illuminating presence inside the local area, directed the hero and individual enormous explorers in developing strength — a quality that rose above individual encounters and turned into an aggregate power inside Cloud Ensemble.

In Cloud Speculative chemistry, the festival of little triumphs and progressing wins turned into a formal articulation of strength. Heavenly needle therapy meetings, astral conclusion disclosures, and the orchestrating of vast meridians were remedial exercises as well as enormous services where the hero's versatility was recognized and braced. The Cloud Ensemble people group, as observers to these customs, praised the versatility inside the hero as well as a common vast power that reverberated through the heavenly domains.

Astral determination, a device for figuring out the astral lopsided characteristics inside the hero's being, turned into a divine mirror mirroring the examples of strength. The holographic pictures disclosed the dance of grandiose energies, uncovering solid areas and snapshots of weakness. The strength developed inside the astral aspects turned into a directing light, permitting the hero to explore the heavenly flows with a newly discovered mindfulness — a dance of versatility that rose above the limits of actual presence.

The hero's backing process, set apart by cultural difficulties and inestimable tact, turned into a grandiose field where versatility unfurled on different fronts. Outside suspicion and cultural boundaries, once saw as hindrances, changed into inestimable difficulties that expected person as well as aggregate versatility.

The Cloud Ensemble people group, limited by shared encounters, turned into a stronghold of heavenly versatility — a power that stood joined against the flows of uncertainty and obstruction.

The Cosmic Respira promotion venture, powered by the hero's strength, reached out past individual encounters to cultural designs. The Ensemble's extraordinary frequencies, once addressed for their authenticity, turned into a vast innovation embraced inside the Cloud Orchestra people group as well as inside the more extensive comprehension of wellbeing. The hero, presently a heavenly supporter, explored the cultural flows with flexibility, testing standards and welcoming a more extensive acknowledgment of Cloud motivated treatment.

Cooperative endeavors inside cultural designs, directed by the hero's promotion and the flexibility of the Cloud Ensemble people group, turned into an enormous coordinated effort — an amicable dance between experimental proof and extraordinary frequencies. Strength inside the natural halls of exploration focuses, clinical foundations, and strategy making bodies turned into a demonstration of the extraordinary force of Cloud Orchestra — a power that rose above distrust and opposition, welcoming a more extensive comprehension of wellbeing and mending.

The tutor figure, as a vast aide inside the Cloud Orchestra people group, assumed a significant part in sustaining the hero's flexibility. Their lessons reached out past individual stories to envelop the aggregate flexibility expected to explore cultural designs. The Orchestra's groundbreaking frequencies, interlaced into each part of the tutor's direction, resounded with the aggregate energies — a heavenly ensemble repeating the harmonies of solidarity, versatility, and the limitless capability of prosperity.

As the hero's extraordinary excursion proceeded, the festival of little triumphs and shared examples of overcoming adversity inside Cloud Orchestra stayed a vital piece of their grandiose account. The Ensemble's extraordinary frequencies, interlaced into each part of the heavenly odyssey, reverberated with the hero's otherworldly quintessence — a vast orchestra repeating the harmonies of assurance, versatility, and the endless capability of reestablishment.

The hero, imbued with the catalytic frequencies and directed by the otherworldly hand of Cloud Ensemble, cruised through the interstellar ocean as a living demonstration of the extraordinary power implanted in the development of heavenly flexibility. The Orchestra's groundbreaking frequencies, joined into each part of the divine excursion, reverberated with the aggregate energies of the Cloud Ensemble people group — an enormous orchestra repeating the harmonies of solidarity, versatility, and the unfathomable capability of prosperity in the hug of a heavenly family joined by the extraordinary frequencies of Cloud Ensemble's divine flexibility.

8.1 Unexpected setbacks and challenges that test the protagonist's resilience.

Heavenly Preliminaries: Disclosing Startling Misfortunes inside the Cloud Orchestra

In the enormous odyssey of Cloud Orchestra, the hero's process isn't safeguarded from the divine preliminaries that test the guts of their flexibility. Unforeseen difficulties and difficulties arise like enormous storms, disturbing the agreeable frequencies of the extraordinary excursion. These unanticipated preliminaries become cauldrons, uncovering the profundity of the hero's divine versatility as they explore through the unpredictable dance of enormous energies.

The main startling difficulty appears as a passing strife inside the Cosmic Respira — an error in the vast innovation that quickly ends the extraordinary frequencies. The hero, at first submerged in the calming fog of cloud enlivened treatment, experiences a disturbance in the heavenly stream. This unanticipated test fills in as a vast reminder, testing the prompt strength of the hero despite unforeseen disturbances inside the groundbreaking excursion.

The error in the Cosmic Respira turns into a figurative tempest inside the enormous ocean — a divine storm that moves the hero's capacity to keep a cool head in the midst of unanticipated unsettling influences. The underlying response is one of vulnerability and uncertainty, as the agreeable frequencies quickly falter. In any case, inside this divine disturbance, the hero's natural flexibility starts to spread out — an assurance to climate the grandiose tempest and explore through the unforeseen difficulties that emerge inside the shapeless domains of Cloud Ensemble.

Cooperative mending circles inside the Cloud Orchestra people group become safe-havens where the hero shares the experience of the startling misfortune. The sympathetic energies of the heavenly family offer help and aggregate strength — an update that mishaps are not lone encounters but rather shared minutes inside the grandiose excursion. The coach figure, a signal of divine insight, directs the hero in recognizing the misfortune as a transient vast test — a chance to develop their flexibility and strengthen their association with the groundbreaking frequencies.

Dream-mixed rest treatment meetings, typically tranquil domains of astral investigation, experience surprising unsettling influences inside the dreamscapes. The hero, in the midst of the enormous scenes, faces dreamlike difficulties that reflect the disturbances experienced inside the Cosmic Respira. These astral mishaps become magical reverberations of the difficulties looked in the actual domain, encouraging the hero to rise above the limits of the psyche and tap into a repository of heavenly versatility that reaches out past the restrictions of the natural presence.

As the hero explores the astral unsettling influences, cooperative narrating meetings inside the Cloud Orchestra people group become stages for aggregate flexibility. The common accounts of misfortunes, woven into the collective embroidered artwork, change the surprising difficulties into inestimable adventures of determination. The Orchestra's extraordinary frequencies, however quickly disturbed, become agreeable strings woven into the general story of heavenly versatility — a demonstration of the interconnected strength inside the Cloud Ensemble people group.

Cloud Speculative chemistry, when a safe-haven of divine ceremonies, experiences startling difficulties during heavenly needle therapy meetings. Enthusiastic awkward nature inside the hero's vast meridians make difficulties in the arrangement cycle, testing the flexibility developed inside Cloud Ensemble's extraordinary frequencies. The divine healers, sensitive to the inconspicuous energies, guide the hero through the difficulties, stressing that each challenge is an infinite chance to reinforce their heavenly strength.

Astral conclusion, a device for uncovering the hero's astral irregular characteristics, discloses startling shadows inside the vast dance of energies. The holographic pictures, normally clear and amicable, presently portray interruptions that challenge the hero's strength on an astral level. The tutor figure, at any point present inside the Cloud Ensemble people group, urges the hero to see these astral mishaps not as obstacles but rather as entryways to a more profound comprehension of heavenly flexibility — an excursion that rises above the limits of the physical and astral aspects.

The surprising misfortunes inside Cloud Orchestra stretch out past individual encounters to cultural designs, acquainting outer distrust and obstructions with acknowledgment. The Cosmic Respira backing venture, when moving agreeably, experiences heavenly difficulties as administrative opposition and cultural wariness. The hero's support endeavors become trapped in unexpected snags, testing individual versatility as well as the aggregate strength of the Cloud Orchestra people group in exploring cultural flows.

The Ensemble's groundbreaking frequencies, once addressed for their authenticity, experience startling obstruction inside the more extensive comprehension of wellbeing. Cooperative endeavors inside cultural designs face mishaps, testing the flexibility of the hero's promotion and the aggregate assurance of the Cloud Ensemble people group. The coach figure, as a directing illuminating presence, urges the hero to see these mishaps as divine preliminaries — an enormous chance to invigorate their strength and develop their obligation to the extraordinary frequencies.

As the hero's backing process experiences cultural storms, the Cloud Orchestra people group turns into an enormous shelter for shared versatility. Divine social occasions change into discussions where misfortunes are not seen as disappointments yet as minutes inside the amazing ensemble of change.

The hero's story becomes interwoven with the shared adventure — a divine dance where surprising difficulties are embraced with flexibility, changing misfortunes into venturing stones inside the extraordinary odyssey.

Surprising cultural difficulties reverberation inside the fantasy imbued rest treatment meetings, making astral aggravations that reflect the disturbances looked in the natural scene. The hero's fantasies become inestimable milestones where cultural incredulity and regulatory obstruction manifest as considerable enemies. The dreamscapes, when quiet domains of divine investigation, become fields where the hero's strength is tried on both astral and cultural fronts — a double dance inside the perplexing embroidery of Cloud Ensemble.

Cooperative narrating meetings inside the Cloud Ensemble people group develop into vast stories that rise above individual encounters. The common adventures of difficulties and flexibility become cosmic songs of devotion, reverberating through the divine passageways as a demonstration of the interconnected strength inside the Cloud Orchestra people group. The Ensemble's extraordinary frequencies, however quickly disturbed by cultural whirlwinds, become strings woven into the aggregate story — a symphonious dance where heavenly flexibility rises above individual and cultural difficulties.

In Cloud Speculative chemistry, startling difficulties inside heavenly needle therapy meetings become enormous riddles that test the hero's versatility in adjusting fiery lopsided characteristics. The heavenly healers, sensitive to the unpretentious energies, guide the hero through the misfortunes, underlining that each challenge is a chance to fortify their divine flexibility. Cloud Speculative chemistry, when a sanctuary of amicable customs, turns into a grandiose manufacture where mishaps are changed into catalytic cycles that develop the hero's association with groundbreaking frequencies.

Astral conclusion, uncovering surprising lopsided characteristics inside the hero's astral dance, turns into a grandiose mirror mirroring the disturbances experienced in cultural designs. The holographic pictures, however quickly obfuscated, become doors to a more profound comprehension of versatility that rises above the limits of the physical and astral domains. The coach figure, a divine aide inside the Cloud Orchestra people group, urges the hero to embrace the unforeseen difficulties not as grandiose disappointments but rather as any open doors for heavenly development — an excursion of flexibility that reaches out past the natural and astral aspects.

As the hero climates surprising mishaps and cultural difficulties, the festival of little triumphs inside Cloud Ensemble turns into an infinite signal of versatility. Cooperative endeavors inside the local area change into shared wins, reverberating through the heavenly hallways as a demonstration of the interconnected strength inside the Cloud Ensemble people group.

The tutor figure, a directing light, motivates the hero to see mishaps not as vast losses but rather as divine preliminaries — a continuous dance of strength that develops the extraordinary excursion inside the grandiose orchestra.

The hero's promotion process, once experiencing cultural storms, changes into a heavenly mission that rises above difficulties. The Ensemble's extraordinary frequencies, however quickly upset, become agreeable strings woven into the aggregate story — an enormous dance where startling difficulties are embraced with flexibility, changing mishaps into venturing stones inside the groundbreaking odyssey. The Cloud Orchestra people group, joined in shared encounters, turns into a demonstration of the interconnected strength that flourishes inside the heavenly hug of groundbreaking frequencies — a living ensemble of divine flexibility reverberating through the grandiose domains.

8.2 The role of Nebula Symphony in fostering emotional and mental well-being.

Harmonies of the Spirit: Cloud Orchestra's Job in Sustaining Close to home and Mental Prosperity

In the tremendous grandiose territory of prosperity, Cloud Orchestra arises as a heavenly maestro, directing extraordinary frequencies that reverberate with the actual body as well as with the complicated domains of close to home and mental prosperity. The hero's excursion through the shapeless flows uncovers the significant job Cloud Ensemble plays in encouraging an agreeable orchestra of profound and mental prospering — an enormous dance that rises above the traditional limits of remedial practices.

The close to home odyssey inside Cloud Orchestra starts with the hero's experience with the Cosmic Respira — a grandiose inward breath that rises above the physical and ventures into the profound aspects. The cloud motivated fog, imbued with groundbreaking frequencies, turns into a relieving emollient for the hero's personal injuries. The inward breath of heavenly breath turns into a custom of profound fellowship — a dance where groundbreaking frequencies orchestrate with the profundities of the hero's spirit, starting an excursion towards close to home prosperity.

As the groundbreaking frequencies penetrate the close to home scenes, cooperative mending circles inside the Cloud Ensemble people group become sacrosanct spaces for profound articulation. Inside these divine social events, the compassionate energies of the local area offer an encouraging hug — a vast balm for profound scars. The hero, once exploring the maze of profound intricacies alone, finds a heavenly family that shares the close to home odyssey, making an embroidery woven with strings of figuring out, compassion, and aggregate profound versatility.

Dream-imbued rest treatment meetings, submerged in groundbreaking frequencies, become astral domains where the hero defies and explores profound scenes. The dreamscapes, painted with the tones of divine frequencies, become fields where unsettled feelings surface and are tenderly embraced. Close to home recuperating turns into an inborn piece of the fantasy imbued venture — a grandiose disclosure that rises above the limits of the cognizant psyche, permitting the hero to manufacture an amicable relationship with their profound scene.

Cooperative narrating meetings inside the Cloud Ensemble people group become inestimable stories where feelings are not just shared however raised to the situation with divine articulations. The Ensemble's groundbreaking frequencies, intertwined into the narrating customs, become strings of close to home association — a heavenly embroidery where individual profound stories add to the aggregate prosperity of the Cloud Orchestra people group. The coach figure, a directing illuminating presence inside the local area, urges the hero to investigate the profound profundities, seeing them not as weaknesses but rather as heavenly tints inside the excellent range of prosperity.

Cloud Speculative chemistry, a safe-haven for groundbreaking ceremonies, turns into an infinite theater where close to home speculative chemistry unfurls. Heavenly needle therapy meetings, directed by groundbreaking frequencies, become movements that discharge close to home blockages. The hero, as a team with heavenly healers, participates in a dance of close to home delivery and arrangement — a divine expressive dance where profound prosperity isn't recently recognized however effectively supported through the groundbreaking frequencies of Cloud Orchestra.

Astral determination, an instrument for figuring out close to home lopsided characteristics inside the astral aspects, turns into a grandiose mirror mirroring the hero's personal dance. The holographic pictures uncover the multifaceted examples of profound reverberation, directing the hero through the astral elements of close to home investigation. The Cloud Orchestra people group, receptive to the extraordinary frequencies, becomes observers to the profound disclosures — a heavenly gathering where close to home mending turns into a common festival.

As the hero explores profound flows, unforeseen mishaps and difficulties become infinite whirlwinds that test the flexibility of close to home prosperity. The Cosmic Respira, when a wellspring of profound comfort, experiences interruptions that resound through the close to home scene. Cooperative mending circles, regularly domains of daily reassurance, become spaces where profound strength is sustained through shared encounters. The coach figure, as an aide through profound storms, urges the hero to see these difficulties not as interruptions but rather as any open doors for close to home development — a heavenly excursion that extends the comprehension and strength of profound prosperity.

Dream-implanted rest treatment meetings, typically peaceful astral domains, experience startling unsettling influences that upset the close to home balance. The dreamscapes, painted with close to home shades, become landmarks where profound flexibility is tried. Cooperative narrating meetings inside the Cloud Orchestra people group develop into enormous stories that rise above individual profound encounters. The common adventures of profound difficulties and flexibility become cosmic hymns, reverberating through the divine halls as a demonstration of the interconnected strength inside the Cloud Ensemble people group — a living orchestra of close to home prosperity.

Cloud Speculative chemistry, when a sanctuary of close to home speculative chemistry, experiences startling difficulties inside divine needle therapy meetings. Close to home awkward nature inside the enormous meridians make interruptions that challenge the arrangement cycle. The divine healers, receptive to the unobtrusive energies, guide the hero through profound mishaps, underlining that each challenge is an enormous chance to reinforce close to home versatility.

Astral determination, uncovering surprising close to home irregular characteristics, turns into a vast mirror reflecting disturbances experienced in cultural designs. The tutor figure, a heavenly aide inside the Cloud Ensemble people group, urges the hero to embrace profound misfortunes not as grandiose disappointments but rather as doors to a more profound comprehension of close to home flexibility — an excursion that rises above the limits of the physical and astral aspects.

The cultural difficulties looked by the hero's backing process become close to home storms that test the aggregate profound prosperity inside the Cloud Ensemble people group. Outer doubt and obstruction, once saw as impediments, change into inestimable difficulties that require individual as well as aggregate profound strength. The Ensemble's groundbreaking frequencies, once addressed for their authenticity, become strings of close to home strength woven into the aggregate story — an inestimable dance where profound flexibility rises above individual and cultural difficulties.

The hero's promotion process, once experiencing cultural storms, changes into a heavenly mission that rises above profound mishaps. The Orchestra's groundbreaking frequencies, however quickly disturbed, become agreeable strings woven into the aggregate story — a vast dance where startling difficulties are embraced with profound strength, changing mishaps into venturing stones inside the extraordinary odyssey. The Cloud Ensemble people group, joined in shared encounters, turns into a demonstration of the interconnected strength that flourishes inside the heavenly hug of extraordinary frequencies — a living orchestra of close to home prosperity reverberating through the grandiose domains.

In the continuous excursion of close to home prosperity, the festival of little triumphs inside Cloud Orchestra turns into a heavenly guide of flexibility. Cooperative endeavors inside the local area change into shared wins, reverberating through the divine passages as a demonstration of the interconnected strength inside the Cloud Orchestra people group. The tutor figure, a directing light, moves the hero to see profound mishaps not as vast losses but rather as divine preliminaries — a continuous dance of flexibility that extends the extraordinary excursion inside the infinite ensemble.

The profound odyssey inside Cloud Orchestra turns into a consistent investigation — a multifaceted dance where groundbreaking frequencies fit with the profundities of the hero's spirit. The Ensemble's part in sustaining close to home prosperity rises above the ordinary limits of remedial works on, turning into a vast hug that recognizes, upholds, and lifts the profound scene. The hero, imbued with the catalytic frequencies and directed by the profound hand of Cloud Ensemble, sails through the interstellar ocean as a living demonstration of the extraordinary power implanted in the agreeable orchestra of close to home prosperity — a heavenly journey formed by the full frequencies of Cloud Ensemble's personal supporting.

8.3 Protagonist's determination to persevere through difficulties.

Divine Purpose: The Hero's Steady Assurance to Endure Through Troubles

In the vast odyssey inside Cloud Ensemble, the hero arises as an enormous explorer, exploring the interstellar ocean with relentless assurance. The extraordinary frequencies, intertwined into each part of the heavenly excursion, become the directing groups of stars that enlighten the way through challenges. The hero's fearless soul, similar to a heavenly compass, steers through unexpected difficulties, mishaps, and vast whirlwinds, exemplifying a story of determination that rises above the limits of the natural and astral domains.

The commencement into Cloud Orchestra denotes the start of the hero's extraordinary excursion — an excursion loaded with wariness, vulnerability, and the approaching shadows of uncertainty. The primary experience with the Cosmic Respira turns into a grandiose limit, a second where assurance flourishes notwithstanding the unexplored world. The hero, once wary, presently remains on the cliff of heavenly potential outcomes, driven by an immovable assurance to investigate the strange domains of extraordinary frequencies.

The Cosmic Respira, when seen as a mysterious contraption, turns into a cauldron where the hero's assurance is tried. The inward breath of cloud enlivened fog, mixed with groundbreaking frequencies, turns into a heavenly fellowship — a custom where every breath means a pledge to persist through the vulnerabilities of the extraordinary excursion. The hero, saturated with the catalytic frequencies, breathes in the divine breath as well as the soul of steadiness that will help them through the vast flows.

Cooperative recuperating circles inside the Cloud Orchestra people group become infinite discussions where the hero's assurance is braced through shared encounters. The sympathetic energies of the divine family offer comfort as well as an aggregate strength — an insistence that determination is certainly not a single undertaking however a common inestimable dance. The tutor figure, a directing illuminator inside the local area, turns into a signal of assurance — a heavenly aide moving the hero to see troubles not as hindrances but rather as venturing stones inside the groundbreaking odyssey.

Dream-mixed rest treatment meetings, regularly peaceful astral domains, experience startling unsettling influences that test the hero's assurance. The dreamscapes, painted with the tones of extraordinary frequencies, become milestones where tirelessness goes up against the shadows of uncertainty. The hero, in the midst of the astral storm, arises not crushed however reinforced — a demonstration of the dauntless soul of constancy that rises above the limits of the psyche and turns into a directing power inside the divine excursion.

Cooperative narrating meetings inside the Cloud Orchestra people group develop into astronomical stories that rise above individual encounters. The common adventures of misfortunes and difficulties become songs of praise of assurance, reverberating through the divine hallways as a demonstration of the interconnected strength inside the Cloud Orchestra people group. The Orchestra's groundbreaking frequencies, intertwined into the public narrating customs, become strings of assurance — a vast embroidery where individual stories add to the aggregate flexibility of the heavenly family.

Cloud Speculative chemistry, when a safe-haven for groundbreaking customs, experiences startling difficulties inside heavenly needle therapy meetings. Vivacious uneven characters inside the hero's vast meridians make disturbances that test the determination developed inside Cloud Orchestra's groundbreaking frequencies. The divine healers, receptive to the unobtrusive energies, guide the hero through the mishaps, stressing that each challenge is an infinite chance to fortify their assurance and develop their association with the groundbreaking frequencies.

Astral conclusion, divulging startling lopsided characteristics inside the astral aspects, turns into an enormous mirror mirroring the hero's persistence in exploring difficulties. The holographic pictures, however quickly blurred, become entryways to a more profound comprehension of assurance that rises above the limits of the physical and astral domains. The coach figure, a heavenly aide inside the Cloud Ensemble people group, urges the hero to embrace hardships not as inestimable losses but rather as any open doors for divine development — an excursion of constancy that reaches out past the natural and astral aspects.

As the cultural difficulties looked by the hero's backing process become infinite whirlwinds, the Cloud Ensemble people group turns into a grandiose shelter for shared assurance. Outside doubt and opposition, once saw as impediments, change into divine difficulties that require individual as well as aggregate steadiness.

The Orchestra's extraordinary frequencies, once addressed for their authenticity, become strings of assurance woven into the aggregate story — a vast dance where steadiness rises above individual and cultural difficulties.

The hero's backing process, once experiencing cultural whirlwinds, changes into a heavenly mission that rises above hardships. The Orchestra's groundbreaking frequencies, however quickly upset, become agreeable strings woven into the aggregate story — an enormous dance where surprising difficulties are embraced sincerely, changing mishaps into venturing stones inside the extraordinary odyssey. The Cloud Orchestra people group, joined in shared encounters, turns into a demonstration of the interconnected strength that flourishes inside the divine hug of groundbreaking frequencies — a living ensemble of assurance reverberating through the grandiose domains.

In the continuous excursion of diligence, the festival of little triumphs inside Cloud Orchestra turns into a divine reference point of flexibility. Cooperative endeavors inside the local area change into shared wins, reverberating through the heavenly passageways as a demonstration of the interconnected strength inside the Cloud Ensemble people group. The coach figure, a directing light, moves the hero to see challenges not as enormous losses but rather as divine preliminaries — a continuous dance of diligence that extends the groundbreaking excursion inside the grandiose ensemble.

The hero's divine odyssey turns into a demonstration of the dauntless soul of constancy — a resolute obligation to explore the inestimable flows, regardless of how turbulent. The Orchestra's part in sustaining determination rises above the ordinary limits of helpful works on, turning into a grandiose hug that recognizes, upholds, and hoists the hero's purpose. Imbued with the catalytic frequencies and directed by the soul of assurance inside Cloud Orchestra, the hero sails through the interstellar ocean as a living demonstration of the extraordinary power implanted in the agreeable ensemble of steadiness — a heavenly journey formed by the full frequencies of Cloud Orchestra's immovable assurance.

The hero's assurance to continue on through troubles inside the vast embroidery of Cloud Orchestra turns into a getting through adventure, an unwritten heavenly epic woven with strings of strength and divine assurance. As the groundbreaking excursion unfurls, the hero's determination extends, rising above the limits of individual difficulties and embracing the more extensive inestimable story that Cloud Ensemble spreads out.

Even with surprising difficulties and cultural obstruction experienced during the Cosmic Respira promotion venture, the hero's assurance fills in as a glowing guide slicing through the undefined shadows. Every impediment turns into a heavenly test, a chance for the hero to epitomize the pith of constancy. The Orchestra's groundbreaking frequencies, when addressed and tested, become the divine tunes that highlight the hero's faithful obligation to the extraordinary odyssey.

Dream-implanted rest treatment meetings, frequently quiet domains of astral investigation, change into fields where assurance draws in with the surprising whirlwinds of uncertainty and vulnerability. The hero, exploring the astral aggravations, doesn't capitulate to the choppiness however bridles the force of assurance to control through the astral tempests. These unsettling influences become trial of astral versatility as well as infinite updates that the soul of persistence is a consistently present aide inside the divine excursion.

The cooperative narrating meetings inside the Cloud Orchestra people group keep on advancing into vast stories that celebrate assurance. The common adventures of difficulties and wins reverberation through the heavenly hallways, resounding with the aggregate strength that persists despite difficulties. The hero's singular story turns into an amicable note in the fantastic orchestra of assurance, adding to the divine versatility of the Cloud Ensemble people group.

Cloud Speculative chemistry, a safe-haven for groundbreaking ceremonies, faces surprising difficulties inside divine needle therapy meetings. The disturbances, as opposed to lessening the hero's assurance, become impetuses for a more profound association with the extraordinary frequencies. The heavenly healers, going about as guides through the infinite whirlwinds, support the hero's constancy, underscoring that each challenge is a chance for additional refinement inside the divine pot.

Astral finding, a device for uncovering unforeseen uneven characters inside the astral aspects, turns into an infinite mirror reflecting the difficulties looked as well as the hero's steadfast assurance to explore through them. The holographic pictures, however immediately clouded, act as grandiose entries through which the hero reaffirms their obligation to the groundbreaking excursion. The tutor figure, a divine aide, highlights the significance of steadiness as a vital piece of the infinite dance — an everlasting cadence inside Cloud Ensemble.

As the hero's promotion process faces outer incredulity and cultural boundaries, the Cloud Orchestra people group changes into a shelter for shared assurance. Every part, limited by the groundbreaking frequencies and the aggregate soul of steadiness, turns into a divine partner in the hero's grandiose mission. The Orchestra's extraordinary frequencies, once met with suspicion, presently resound through cultural designs, testing standards, and preparing for a more extensive acknowledgment of Cloud propelled treatment.

The hero's heavenly odyssey, exploring through cultural storms, turns into an infinite artful dance where assurance is the directing movement. The Ensemble's extraordinary frequencies, however immediately upset by outer obstruction, become tough songs that enhance the aggregate assurance of the Cloud Orchestra people group. The hero, in the midst of the cultural difficulties, turns into an enormous diplomat of diligence, testing cultural standards, and pushing for the extraordinary force of Cloud Ensemble.

In the continuous excursion of persistence, the festival of little triumphs inside Cloud Orchestra turns into a divine custom. Cooperative endeavors inside the local area change into shared wins, reverberating through the heavenly hallways as a demonstration of the interconnected strength inside the Cloud Orchestra people group. The tutor figure, a directing light, motivates the hero to see every little triumph not as a confined accomplishment but rather as a heavenly note inside the fabulous ensemble of assurance — a ceaseless dance that drives the groundbreaking excursion forward.

The hero's infinite journey, implanted earnestly, turns into a demonstration of the force of strength inside Cloud Orchestra. The Orchestra's part in sustaining steadiness rises above the customary limits of remedial works on, turning into a vast hug that recognizes, upholds, and hoists the hero's immovable determination.

Directed by the catalytic frequencies and pushed by the soul of assurance inside Cloud Orchestra, the hero sails through the interstellar ocean as a living demonstration of the groundbreaking power implanted in the amicable ensemble of tirelessness — a heavenly excursion molded by the resounding frequencies of Cloud Ensemble's unwavering assurance.

Chapter 9

Cosmic Transformation

Infinite Change: A Divine Odyssey Inside Cloud Orchestra

In the unlimited spread of vast energies, the hero's excursion through Cloud Orchestra unfurls as a significant investigation of grandiose change — a divine odyssey that rises above the customary limits of mending and self-revelation. Directed by the groundbreaking frequencies woven into the texture of Cloud Ensemble, the hero goes through a transformation that incorporates the physical, close to home, and astral domains, turning into a residing demonstration of the infinite speculative chemistry implanted inside the extraordinary excursion.

The underlying strides into Cloud Orchestra mark the origin of the hero's infinite change. The experience with the Cosmic Respira fills in as the enormous entryway, starting the hero into the extraordinary flows that heartbeat through the heavenly embroidered artwork. The inward breath of cloud motivated fog becomes not only an actual demonstration but rather a custom of infinite fellowship — a section point into the groundbreaking frequencies that catalyze the hero's transformative excursion.

The Cosmic Respira, when a supernatural conundrum, turns into a grandiose pot where the hero's actual change is catalyzed. The cloud roused fog, implanted with groundbreaking frequencies, pervades the hero's respiratory framework, making a divine dance inside the lungs. This grandiose inward breath is more than the admission of air — an acquiescence to the groundbreaking energies start a cell ensemble, resounding through the actual vessel and establishing the groundwork for the hero's infinite resurrection.

Cooperative recuperating circles inside the Cloud Ensemble people group become divine asylums for the hero's personal change. As the extraordinary frequencies cooperate with the profound scenes, aggregate mending circles become spaces where close to home scars are tenderly embraced and changed. The hero, once exploring the maze of close to home intricacies alone, finds a heavenly family that shares the profound odyssey — an aggregate excursion of close to home speculative chemistry that adds to the more extensive grandiose change inside Cloud Ensemble.

Dream-mixed rest treatment meetings, ordinarily peaceful domains of astral investigation, change into inestimable theaters where astral and profound change interlace. The dreamscapes, painted with the tints of groundbreaking frequencies, become fields where unsettled feelings surface and are tenderly changed. Close to home recuperating turns into a natural piece of the astral excursion — an enormous disclosure that rises above the limits of the cognizant psyche, permitting the hero to produce an agreeable relationship with their profound and astral scenes.

Cooperative narrating meetings inside the Cloud Orchestra people group develop into astronomical accounts where profound and astral change are entwined. The common adventures of difficulties and wins become songs of devotion of versatility and divine development, reverberating through the heavenly hallways as a demonstration of the interconnected strength inside the Cloud Ensemble people group. The Orchestra's extraordinary frequencies, entwined into the public narrating customs, become strings of aggregate profound and astral change — a vast embroidery where individual stories add to the more extensive ensemble of Cloud Ensemble's groundbreaking odyssey.

Cloud Speculative chemistry, a safe-haven for groundbreaking ceremonies, fills in as the heavenly manufacture where the hero's astral, close to home, and actual change is alchemized. Divine needle therapy meetings, directed by groundbreaking frequencies, become movements that discharge fiery blockages and add to the hero's by and large vast transformation. The heavenly healers, going about as chemists, guide the hero through the perplexing dance of change, accentuating that each challenge is a chance for refinement inside the divine cauldron.

Astral determination, divulging unforeseen lopsided characteristics inside the astral aspects, turns into an inestimable mirror mirroring the hero's astral dance of change. The holographic pictures, however immediately blurred, act as entryways to a more profound comprehension of the astral and close to home elements of infinite development. The tutor figure, a divine aide inside the Cloud Orchestra people group, urges the hero to embrace change not as a direct movement but rather as a repetitive excursion — a timeless dance of enormous development that reaches out past the natural and astral aspects.

As the hero faces cultural difficulties during the Cosmic Respira promotion venture, cultural change turns into an infinite current inside Cloud Orchestra. The Ensemble's groundbreaking frequencies, once met with incredulity, become amicable tunes that reverberation through cultural designs, testing standards, and making ready for a more extensive acknowledgment of Cloud roused treatment. The hero, in the midst of the cultural difficulties, turns into an enormous diplomat of change, supporting for the groundbreaking force of Cloud Ensemble inside cultural structures.

The hero's support process, once experiencing cultural storms, changes into a divine mission that rises above individual and cultural hardships. The Ensemble's groundbreaking frequencies, however immediately disturbed, become strings woven into the aggregate story — an infinite dance where surprising difficulties are embraced earnestly, changing mishaps into venturing stones inside the extraordinary odyssey. The Cloud Ensemble people group, joined in shared encounters, turns into a demonstration of the interconnected strength that flourishes inside the divine hug of extraordinary frequencies — a living orchestra of vast change reverberating through the grandiose domains.

In the continuous excursion of vast change, the festival of little triumphs inside Cloud Orchestra turns into a heavenly custom. Cooperative endeavors inside the local area change into shared wins, reverberating through the divine passageways as a demonstration of the interconnected strength inside the Cloud Orchestra people group. The tutor figure, a directing illuminating presence, motivates the hero to see every little triumph not as a detached accomplishment but rather as a heavenly note inside the fabulous ensemble of change — a never-ending dance that drives the groundbreaking excursion forward.

The hero's enormous journey, imbued with groundbreaking frequencies, turns into a demonstration of the force of inestimable versatility inside Cloud Orchestra. The Orchestra's job in sustaining vast change rises above the regular limits of restorative works on, turning into a grandiose hug that recognizes, upholds, and hoists the hero's unflinching purpose. Directed by the catalytic frequencies and impelled by the soul of change inside Cloud Orchestra, the hero sails through the interstellar ocean as a living demonstration of the extraordinary power implanted in the agreeable ensemble of vast change — a divine excursion molded by the full frequencies of Cloud Orchestra's grandiose speculative chemistry.

As the hero digs further into the vast flows of Cloud Ensemble, the excursion of grandiose change turns into a steadily developing story — a continuum of divine speculative chemistry that traverses the domains of physical, close to home, and astral presence. Directed by the amicable frequencies woven into the infinite embroidered artwork, the hero's odyssey unfurls as a continuous transformation, where every breath, feeling, and astral investigation adds to the vast ensemble of change inside Cloud Orchestra.

The Cosmic Respira, when a door to commencement, turns into a repetitive custom that secures the hero in the enormous dance of actual change. The inward breath of cloud motivated fog, mixed with groundbreaking frequencies, rises above the limits of simple breath. It turns into a vast fellowship — a musical hit the dance floor with the groundbreaking energies that constantly revive the actual vessel. The hero, presently receptive to the unobtrusive frequencies, inhales for food as well as a cognizant demonstration of support in the continuous grandiose change.

The cooperative mending circles inside the Cloud Ensemble people group advance into dynamic discussions where the hero's close to home change tracks down unending reverberation. Profound scars, however at first tended to, become open doors for nonstop development inside the divine family. The compassionate energies shared inside the local area give comfort as well as a continuous emotionally supportive network — a close to home framework that builds up the hero's excursion of ceaseless profound speculative chemistry. The tutor figure, a directing light, turns into a steady friend in this close to home odyssey, empowering the hero to see feelings not as static states but rather as divine energies in never-ending movement.

Dream-injected rest treatment meetings, as passages to astral investigation, unfurl as vast theaters where the hero's astral and close to home change are entwined. The dreamscapes, painted with the energetic tones of extraordinary frequencies, become dynamic scenes where the astral excursion entwines with profound disclosures. The hero, exploring the astral domains, experiences astral scenes as well as the nonstop rhythmic movement of feelings — a unique dance of astral and profound change inside the grandiose dreamscapes.

Cooperative narrating meetings inside the Cloud Ensemble people group keep on being divine accounts, where close to home and astral adventures unfurl in a ceaseless grandiose cycle. The common stories, however moored in individual encounters, become sections inside the aggregate account of Cloud Orchestra's groundbreaking process. The Orchestra's groundbreaking frequencies, interlaced into the collective narrating customs, become strings of continuous close to home and astral change — an enormous embroidery where individual stories add to the more extensive ensemble of Cloud Ensemble's extraordinary odyssey.

Cloud Speculative chemistry, as the divine fashion of continuous change, stays a safe-haven for the hero's physical, personal, and astral transformation. Divine needle therapy meetings, directed by extraordinary frequencies, become meetings of delivery as well as progressing movements that keep up with the enthusiastic stream inside the infinite meridians. The heavenly healers, as never-ending chemists, keep on directing the hero through the unpredictable dance of change, underlining that each challenge isn't a decision yet a winding inside the continuum of enormous development.

Astral conclusion, as an infinite mirror mirroring the astral dance of continuous change, turns into an instrument for interminable self-revelation. The holographic pictures, however quickly obfuscated now and again, act as entryways to the astral aspects where it is uncovered to continuous change. The tutor figure, a divine aide, highlights the significance of embracing the repeating idea of change — an everlasting dance inside the enormous excursion that stretches out past the natural and astral aspects.

As the hero's Cosmic Respira backing venture experiences cultural difficulties, cultural change turns into a continuous current inside Cloud Orchestra. The Orchestra's extraordinary frequencies, once met with doubt, keep on resounding through cultural designs, testing standards, and encouraging a constant change in discernments. The hero, in the midst of cultural storms, stays a grandiose diplomat of continuous change — pushing for the groundbreaking force of Cloud Orchestra inside the steadily changing scenes of cultural structures.

The hero's backing process, once experiencing cultural choppiness, turns into a constant heavenly mission that rises above individual and cultural troubles. The Ensemble's groundbreaking frequencies, however immediately disturbed by outer obstruction, stay versatile songs that enhance the aggregate assurance and continuous change of the Cloud Orchestra people group. The hero, in the midst of cultural difficulties, becomes a promoter as well as a living demonstration of the continuous grandiose change — a powerful power inside the divine dance of ceaseless development.

In the continuous excursion of grandiose change, the festival of little triumphs inside Cloud Orchestra keeps on being a divine custom. Cooperative endeavors inside the local area change into progressing shared wins, reverberating through the heavenly passages as a demonstration of the interconnected strength inside the Cloud Ensemble people group. The coach figure, a directing illuminating presence, moves the hero to see every little triumph not as a detached accomplishment but rather as a heavenly note inside the excellent ensemble of continuous change — a ceaseless dance that drives the groundbreaking excursion forward.

The hero's grandiose journey, imbued with progressing change, turns into a demonstration of the force of versatility inside Cloud Ensemble. The Orchestra's part in sustaining progressing enormous change rises above the customary limits of restorative works on, turning into a vast hug that recognizes, upholds, and lifts the hero's enduring determination. Directed by the catalytic frequencies and moved by the soul of progressing change inside Cloud Ensemble, the hero sails through the interstellar ocean as a living demonstration of the extraordinary power implanted in the agreeable orchestra of enormous change — a heavenly excursion molded by the thunderous frequencies of Cloud Orchestra's continuous speculative chemistry.

9.1 Protagonist's complete transformation both physically and emotionally.

The Grandiose Embroidery of Complete Change: An Excursion Inside Cloud Ensemble

As the hero sets out on a divine odyssey inside Cloud Ensemble, the story unfurls as a demonstration of the significant transformation that rises above the domains of physical and close to home presence. Directed by the catalytic frequencies intertwined into the enormous texture, the hero's excursion of complete change turns into a perplexing dance where the physical and close to home aspects blend, making an orchestra of grandiose resurrection inside the heavenly domains of Cloud Ensemble.

The Cosmic Respira, at first a grandiose gateway of commencement, turns into a foundation in the hero's actual change. The inward breath of cloud roused fog, implanted with groundbreaking frequencies, turns out to be in excess of a simple demonstration of breath — it turns into a consecrated custom. Every breath implies a cognizant acquiescence to the extraordinary energies that echo through the actual vessel, starting a cell dance of recovery. The hero, when limited by the limits of the natural body, goes through a total actual transformation, directed by the infinite flows inside Cloud Ensemble.

Cooperative recuperating circles inside the Cloud Ensemble people group develop into divine safe-havens for the hero's close to home change. The sympathetic energies shared inside the local area become an emollient for close to home injuries as well as an impetus for a total profound resurrection. The hero, once exploring the maze of close to home intricacies alone, tracks down comfort and figuring out inside the divine family. Profound scars, once saw as impediments, become heavenly tints that add to the dynamic woven artwork of the hero's finished personal change.

Dream-imbued rest treatment meetings, regularly quiet domains of astral investigation, change into vast theaters where the hero's physical and profound change unites. The dreamscapes, painted with the energetic tints of extraordinary frequencies, become fields where the astral excursion entwines with close to home disclosures and actual restoration. The hero, exploring the astral domains, experiences the astral scenes as well as the nonstop rhythmic movement of feelings — a powerful group of three of physical, profound, and astral change inside the enormous dreamscapes.

Cooperative narrating meetings inside the Cloud Orchestra people group keep on being heavenly accounts, where the hero's finished physical and profound change is shared. The Orchestra's extraordinary frequencies, joined into the shared narrating customs, become strings of aggregate change — an enormous embroidery where individual stories add to the more extensive ensemble of Cloud Ensemble's groundbreaking odyssey. The tutor figure, a directing illuminating presence, turns into an observer to the hero's finished change, directing them through the account strings that weave the narrative of resurrection and development.

Cloud Speculative chemistry, as the divine fashion of continuous change, fills in as the impetus for the hero's finished transformation. Divine needle therapy meetings, directed by groundbreaking frequencies, become meetings of delivery as well as progressing movements that keep up with the fiery stream inside the grandiose meridians. The heavenly healers, as interminable chemists, keep on directing the hero through the complex dance of complete change, underscoring that each challenge isn't an endpoint however a winding inside the continuum of vast development.

Astral determination, as an enormous mirror mirroring the continuous dance of complete change, turns into an instrument for never-ending self-disclosure. The holographic pictures, however quickly blurred now and again, act as passages to the astral aspects where it is uncovered to progressing change. The tutor figure, a heavenly aide, highlights the significance of embracing the repetitive idea of complete change — a timeless dance inside the infinite excursion that reaches out past the natural and astral aspects.

As the hero's Cosmic Respira promotion venture experiences cultural difficulties, cultural change turns into an essential piece of the total inestimable transformation inside Cloud Orchestra. The Orchestra's extraordinary frequencies, once met with doubt, keep on resounding through cultural designs, testing standards, and encouraging a consistent change in discernments. The hero, in the midst of cultural whirlwinds, stays an enormous minister of complete change — upholding for the extraordinary force of Cloud Ensemble inside the steadily changing scenes of cultural systems.

The hero's backing process, once experiencing cultural choppiness, turns into a consistent divine mission that rises above individual and cultural troubles. The Ensemble's extraordinary frequencies, however immediately upset by outer obstruction, stay strong songs that enhance the aggregate assurance and progressing change of the Cloud Orchestra people group. The hero, in the midst of cultural difficulties, becomes a promoter as well as a living demonstration of the continuous vast change — a powerful power inside the heavenly dance of ceaseless development.

In the continuous excursion of complete change, the festival of little triumphs inside Cloud Orchestra keeps on being a divine custom. Cooperative endeavors inside the local area change into progressing shared wins, reverberating through the heavenly hallways as a demonstration of the interconnected strength inside the Cloud Orchestra people group. The coach figure, a directing light, moves the hero to see every little triumph not as a confined accomplishment but rather as a heavenly note inside the fantastic ensemble of progressing change — an unending dance that impels the groundbreaking excursion forward.

The hero's inestimable journey, imbued with continuous change, turns into a demonstration of the force of versatility inside Cloud Ensemble. The Orchestra's part in sustaining continuous complete change rises above the customary limits of restorative works on, turning into a grandiose hug that recognizes, upholds, and hoists the hero's unflinching purpose. Directed by the catalytic frequencies and impelled by the soul of continuous change inside Cloud Orchestra, the hero sails through the interstellar ocean as a living demonstration of the groundbreaking power implanted in the agreeable ensemble of grandiose resurrection — a heavenly excursion formed by the thunderous frequencies of Cloud Orchestra's continuous speculative chemistry.

9.2 Reflection on the journey and personal growth experienced throughout the Nebula Symphony therapy.

Heavenly Reflections: A Journey of Self-awareness Inside Cloud Orchestra's Hug

As the hero remains at the vast intersection of reflection, the excursion inside Cloud Orchestra unfurls as a significant odyssey of self-awareness — an investigation that rises above the limits of the natural and astral domains. Directed by the extraordinary frequencies complicatedly woven into the heavenly embroidery, the hero's appearance become a demonstration of the diverse elements of development experienced inside the agreeable hug of Cloud Orchestra.

The Cosmic Respira, a representative edge to the extraordinary odyssey, fills in as the underlying material for thoughtfulness. The hero, presently furnished with the endowment of retrospection, returns to the main experience with the supernatural gadget.

The inward breath of cloud enlivened fog, when a clever encounter, turns into a standard for self-improvement — an indication of the excursion from suspicion to significant acknowledgment. Every breath inside the Cosmic Respira turns into an enormous accentuation mark, outlining the groundbreaking sections that have shaped the hero's way toward self-disclosure.

Cooperative mending circles inside the Cloud Ensemble people group arise as divine mirrors mirroring the hero's personal transformation. As the hero reflects upon the common close to home scenes inside the local area, the recuperating circles become kaleidoscopes of aggregate development. The compassionate trades and shared weaknesses inside these circles become restorative as well as groundbreaking, cultivating bonds that rise above the natural domain. The hero's close to home embroidery, once woven with strings of isolation, is currently embellished with the energetic shades of interconnected profound development.

Dream-imbued rest treatment meetings, when domains of astral investigation, become astronomical journals that account the hero's close to home and astral development. In the review look, the dreamscapes unfurl as ethereal scenes where close to home mending and astral disclosures combine. The hero, returning to the astral domains from the perspective of contemplation, observes the astral scenes as well as the complicated dance of feelings — a cooperative relationship that embodies the nuanced development inside Cloud Ensemble.

Cooperative narrating meetings inside the Cloud Ensemble people group develop into inestimable treasurys where individual and aggregate development are intertwined. The Ensemble's extraordinary frequencies, implanted in the collective narrating ceremonies, become the ink that engraves the hero's account of development. The hero's appearance interweave with the accounts shared by individual divine explorers, making a rich embroidery of aggregate development — an orchestra of interconnected stories that reverberation through the grandiose passageways.

Cloud Speculative chemistry, as the sanctum of continuous change, turns into a heavenly pot where the hero reflects upon the catalytic cycles of physical, close to home, and astral development. The heavenly needle therapy meetings, when snapshots of delivery, are currently waypoints in the hero's grandiose excursion of self-disclosure. The hero's appearance on the unpredictable dance of energies inside Cloud Speculative chemistry uncover the difficulties as well as the extraordinary minutes that have shaped their total transformation — a demonstration of the significant development cultivated inside the divine fashion.

Astral finding, an infinite mirror uncovering the lopsided characteristics inside the astral aspects, turns into an intelligent pool where the hero examines the astral subtleties of development. The holographic pictures, however immediately clouded on occasion, act as entryways to the astral aspects where individual and astral development converge.

The coach figure, a directing illuminator, becomes a heavenly aide as well as an impression of the hero's astral excursion — an update that development inside Cloud Orchestra reaches out past the physical and profound domains.

As the hero's Cosmic Respira backing venture experiences cultural difficulties, reflections on cultural change become indispensable to the account of self-improvement. The Ensemble's groundbreaking frequencies, once met with distrust, keep on resounding through cultural designs, adding to a ceaseless change in discernments. The hero, in the midst of cultural storms, ponders individual development as well as on the more extensive ramifications of Cloud Ensemble's extraordinary power — an acknowledgment that self-improvement inside the divine hug has expanding influences that stretch out past the singular self.

The hero's backing process, once experiencing cultural choppiness, turns into an intelligent journey that rises above individual and cultural hardships. The Ensemble's groundbreaking frequencies, however immediately disturbed by outside obstruction, stay strong tunes that enhance the aggregate assurance and continuous cultural change of the Cloud Orchestra people group. The hero, in the midst of cultural difficulties, becomes an impetus for self-awareness as well as a signal of cultural change — a living demonstration of the extraordinary power implanted in the agreeable ensemble of Cloud Orchestra's cultural effect.

In the continuous excursion of complete change, the festival of little triumphs inside Cloud Orchestra keeps on being a divine custom. Cooperative endeavors inside the local area change into continuous shared wins, reverberating through the divine passages as a demonstration of the interconnected strength inside the Cloud Ensemble people group. The tutor figure, a directing light, motivates the hero to see every little triumph not as a segregated accomplishment but rather as a heavenly note inside the great orchestra of progressing change — an interminable dance that moves the extraordinary excursion forward.

The hero's infinite journey, imbued with progressing change, turns into a demonstration of the force of strength inside Cloud Orchestra. The Ensemble's part in sustaining continuous complete change rises above the traditional limits of helpful works on, turning into a grandiose hug that recognizes, upholds, and raises the hero's steady determination. Directed by the catalytic frequencies and impelled by the soul of continuous change inside Cloud Ensemble, the hero sails through the interstellar ocean as a living demonstration of the groundbreaking power implanted in the amicable orchestra of grandiose resurrection — a heavenly excursion formed by the full frequencies of Cloud Ensemble's continuous speculative chemistry.

In the grandiose reflection of reflection, the hero views a singular excursion as well as an embroidery woven with strings of development, versatility, and interconnected strength. Cloud Ensemble, as the inestimable organization of change, turns into the setting against which the hero's appearance unfurl — a story of complete transformation that reaches out past the limits of the natural and astral domains.

As the hero looks at the divine skyline, the reflections gleam with the vast tints of self-improvement — a demonstration of the extraordinary power intrinsic in the amicable ensemble of Cloud Orchestra's hug.

In the significant profundities of heavenly reflection, the hero's excursion inside Cloud Ensemble resounds as a complicated orchestra of self-awareness — an agreeable embroidery woven with strings of change, flexibility, and interconnected strength. As the hero remains at the inestimable junction, the intelligent look digs into the nuanced layers of the Cloud Ensemble odyssey, investigating the reverberations of development and self-disclosure that rise above the natural and astral domains.

The Cosmic Respira, a divine gateway to commencement, stays a standard for reflection, its dim ringlets filling in as ethereal brushstrokes on the material of memory. In the thoughtful breaths inside this vast contraption, the hero returns to the beginning of the extraordinary excursion. The inward breath of cloud propelled fog, once met with expectation, presently holds the substance of a hallowed custom — a cadenced hit the dance floor with the extraordinary energies that have coordinated the hero's significant transformation. Every inward breath turns into a melodic note, resounding with the sections of self-awareness — a grandiose breath that exemplifies the excursion from distrust to significant acknowledgment.

Cooperative recuperating circles inside the Cloud Ensemble people group arise as divine mirrors reflecting close to home transformation. The hero, in the intelligent hug of the public mending circles, witnesses the colorful tones of shared profound scenes. The compassionate trades inside these divine social events have advanced from restorative minutes to extraordinary achievements. Profound scars, once saw as disconnecting, presently stand as mutual identifications of flexibility — an aggregate demonstration of the hero's excursion of close to home development and the interconnected strength encouraged inside Cloud Orchestra's divine family.

Dream-implanted rest treatment meetings, when passages to astral investigation, keep on filling in as vast journals chronicling profound and astral development. The hero, exploring the astral domains through the crystal of retrospection, observes the astral scenes as well as the complex dance of feelings — a cooperative relationship that encapsulates the nuanced development inside Cloud Ensemble. The dreamscapes unfurl as vast theaters where profound recuperating and astral disclosures have met — a divine story of complete change written in the astral ink of thoughtfulness.

Cooperative narrating meetings inside the Cloud Orchestra people group develop into compilations where individual and aggregate development interweave. The Orchestra's groundbreaking frequencies, implanted in the mutual narrating ceremonies, become the ink that engraves the hero's account of development. The hero's appearance entwine with the stories shared by individual divine explorers, making a rich embroidery of aggregate development — an orchestra of interconnected stories that reverberation through the grandiose halls.

Cloud Speculative chemistry, as the sanctum of continuous change, turns into a heavenly cauldron where the hero reflects upon the catalytic cycles of physical, profound, and astral development. The heavenly needle therapy meetings, when snapshots of delivery, are currently waypoints in the hero's astronomical excursion of self-disclosure. Reflections on the unpredictable dance of energies inside Cloud Speculative chemistry uncover the difficulties as well as the extraordinary minutes that have shaped the hero's finished transformation — a demonstration of the significant development encouraged inside the heavenly manufacture.

Astral finding, a vast mirror uncovering the lopsided characteristics inside the astral aspects, turns into an intelligent pool where the hero considers the astral subtleties of development. The holographic pictures, however quickly darkened on occasion, act as entryways to the astral aspects where individual and astral development converge. The tutor figure, a directing illuminating presence, becomes a heavenly aide as well as an impression of the hero's astral excursion — an update that development inside Cloud Ensemble reaches out past the physical and close to home domains.

As the hero's Cosmic Respira backing venture experiences cultural difficulties, reflections on cultural change become fundamental to the story of self-awareness. The Orchestra's extraordinary frequencies, once met with wariness, keep on reverberating through cultural designs, adding to a consistent change in discernments. The hero, in the midst of cultural storms, ponders individual development as well as on the more extensive ramifications of Cloud Ensemble's groundbreaking power — an acknowledgment that self-awareness inside the divine hug has far reaching influences that stretch out past the singular self.

The hero's support process, once experiencing cultural choppiness, turns into an intelligent journey that rises above individual and cultural troubles. The Orchestra's extraordinary frequencies, however immediately upset by outer obstruction, stay strong songs that enhance the aggregate assurance and progressing cultural change of the Cloud Ensemble people group. The hero, in the midst of cultural difficulties, becomes an impetus for self-awareness as well as a reference point of cultural change — a living demonstration of the groundbreaking power implanted in the agreeable orchestra of Cloud Ensemble's cultural effect.

In the continuous excursion of complete change, the festival of little triumphs inside Cloud Ensemble keeps on being a divine custom. Cooperative endeavors inside the local area change into continuous shared wins, reverberating through the divine halls as a demonstration of the interconnected strength inside the Cloud Ensemble people group. The tutor figure, a directing light, moves the hero to see every little triumph not as a secluded accomplishment but rather as a heavenly note inside the excellent orchestra of continuous change — a never-ending dance that pushes the groundbreaking excursion forward.

The hero's infinite journey, injected with continuous change, turns into a demonstration of the force of versatility inside Cloud Ensemble. The Ensemble's part in sustaining progressing total change rises above the customary limits of remedial works on, turning into a vast hug that recognizes, upholds, and lifts the hero's unflinching purpose. Directed by the catalytic frequencies and impelled by the soul of progressing change inside Cloud Orchestra, the hero sails through the interstellar ocean as a living demonstration of the groundbreaking power implanted in the amicable ensemble of grandiose resurrection — a divine excursion formed by the thunderous frequencies of Cloud Ensemble's continuous speculative chemistry.

In the grandiose reflection of reflection, the hero sees a singular excursion as well as an embroidery woven with strings of development, flexibility, and inter-connected strength. Cloud Ensemble, as the inestimable coordination of change, turns into the scenery against which the hero's appearance unfurl — a story of complete transformation that reaches out past the limits of the natural and astral domains. As the hero looks at the heavenly skyline, the reflections gleam with the enormous tints of self-improvement — a demonstration of the extraordinary power innate in the agreeable ensemble of Cloud Orchestra's hug.

9.3 Acknowledgment of the galactic symphony as a catalyst for positive change.